LOW FODMAP, HIGH FIBER, GLUTEN FREE DIET

A Nutritional Blueprint to Eliminate Abdominal Disorders, Support Gut Health, and Manage Weight

Joe Miller, RD

Copyright Page

Copyright © 2024 Joe Miller, RD

Table of Contents

Copyright Page 2

Table of Contents 3

UNDERSTANDING THE LOW FODMAP DIET 1

How do FODMAPs affect digestion? 4

Benefits of a low FODMAP diet 7

Foods to avoid and foods to include 12

Getting started with the low FODMAP diet ... 17

INCORPORATING HIGH FIBER FOODS 50

High fiber foods that are low in FODMAPs ... 63

How to increase fiber intake gradually 67

Tips for Shopping and Meal Preparation 70

THE GLUTEN-FREE APPROACH 76

Benefits of a gluten-free diet.............................80

Gluten-free grains and their nutritional benefits
....86

How to avoid hidden sources of gluten...........99

Gluten-free baking and cooking tips..............100

LOW FODMAP, HIGH FIBER, GLUTEN FREE
DIET RECIPES FOR BREAKFAST......................108

Roasted stone fruits with vanilla 108

Banana, clementine & mango smoothie.........110

Hash browns with gruyère & pancetta..........111

Mango & passion fruit smoothie 115

Oven-baked egg & chips 116

Sprout & spinach baked eggs 117

Fruit & seed yogurt 120

Instant berry banana slush.................................121

Veggie breakfast bakes 122

Sweet potato pancakes with orange & grapefruit
....123

Cloud eggs...125

Tropical breakfast smoothie 127

Blueberry smoothie recipe 128

Crispy hash browns 130

LOW FODMAP, HIGH FIBER, GLUTEN FREE
DIET RECIPES FOR LUNCH 133

Rustic beans & spinach with garlic yogurt....133

Cumin-spiced chicken with squash................136

Spicy tuna quinoa salad 139

Potato frittata with pepper salsa 141

Air-fryer boiled eggs................................144

Vegan nuggets 145

Prawn & avocado wrap...................................149

Lebanese-style meatballs with mujadara.......151

Tomato, watermelon & feta salad with mint dressing....................................155

Roasted summer vegetable casserole.............156

Bean & quinoa salad with orange...................158

Tuna, avocado & pea salad in Baby Gem lettuce wraps...................................161

Watermelon, prawn & avocado salad............162

Smoked mackerel & beetroot salad with creamy horseradish dressing...................................164

LOW FODMAP, HIGH FIBER, GLUTEN FREE DIET RECIPES FOR DINNER 168

Alu tamatar masala 168

Air-fryer turkey crown 171

Chorizo & chickpea summer stew 173

Poached chicken breast 175

Toddler recipe: Microwave courgette and pea risotto with prawns 177

Fennel, cherry & goat's cheese salad with lentils 179

Vegan Thai green curry 182

Loaded potato skins with speedy baked beans 185

Air-fryer fish & chips 187

Honeyed harissa cod with crispy chickpeas .191

Beef & swede casserole....................................193

Turkey, courgetti & feta burgers.....................196

Cumin-spiced halloumi with corn & tomato slaw 199

Korean clam broth - Jogaetang.......................202

Vibrant spinach, coconut & paneer curry......205

LOW FODMAP, HIGH FIBER, GLUTEN FREE DIET RECIPES FOR SNACKS 210

Sticky roasted parsnips, Chantenay carrots & apples 210

Mexican corn on the cob.................................211

Pickled green beans...213

Perfect sushi rice...216

Black beans & rice 219

Brown-butter basted radishes & asparagus ..220

Crunchy parsnips 222

Spicy cauliflower pilau.....................224

Wilted spinach with nutmeg & garlic 225

Clementine & Port spiced cranberry sauce ...226

Salted caramel parsnips.....................228

Tomato, watermelon & feta salad with mint dressing...230

Pickled carrot & mooli.....................232

Spiced braised red cabbage...................233

LIFESTYLE AND LONG-TERM MANAGEMENT 237

Monitoring symptoms and making adjustments to your diet 237

Long-term benefits of a low FODMAP, high fiber, and gluten-free lifestyle 241

CHAPTER 1
UNDERSTANDING THE LOW FODMAP DIET

FODMAP stands for fermentable oligosaccharides, disaccharides, monosaccharides and polyols.

FODMAPs are specific types of short-chain carbohydrates that some people find difficult to efficiently absorb. They are sugar molecules that are linked together in chains and they are fermentable by the bacteria in your gut. Instead of being absorbed into your bloodstream, they reach the far end of your intestine, where most of your gut bacteria live. Certain bacteria in your digestive tract then start to feed on these carbohydrates, using them for fuel, producing hydrogen gas and causing digestive symptoms in sensitive individuals. FODMAPs also draw liquid into your intestine, which may cause diarrhea.

Although not everyone has a sensitivity to FODMAPs, it is very common among people with irritable bowel syndrome (IBS).

The specific types of carbohydrates that are considered FODMAPs include:

• **Oligosaccharides**, which are found in foods like legumes, wheat, garlic, and onions.

• **Disaccharides**, which are found in dairy products, cane or beet sugar, and malt sugar

• **Monosaccharides**, which include sugars found in fruit, honey, and sugary drinks

• **Polyols**, which are found in some types of fruit, certain vegetables, and sugar-free sweeteners

Common FODMAPs include:

• **Fructose**: a simple sugar found in many fruits and vegetables that also makes up the structure of table sugar and most added sugars

• **Lactose**: a carbohydrate found in dairy products like milk

• **Fructans**: found in many foods, including grains like wheat, spelt, rye and barley

• **Galactans**: found in large amounts in legumes

• **Polyols**: sugar alcohols like xylitol, sorbitol, maltitol, and mannitol. They are found in some fruits and vegetables and often used as sweeteners

Some people experience digestive distress after eating them. Symptoms include:

• Cramping

• Diarrhea

• Constipation

• Stomach bloating

• Gas and flatulence

How do FODMAPs affect digestion?

FODMAP foods contain sugars and polyols known to cause GI symptoms, like gas and diarrhea. They may be poorly absorbed in the GI tract and begin to ferment in the intestines. This is especially true for people with IBS and other GI disorders.

How does a FODMAP diet work?

It is important to note that low FODMAP diets are restrictive and should be temporary, lasting only 4–6 weeks. They aim to identify whether specific foods trigger symptoms.

A low FODMAP diet involves three phases. Monash University, which first proposed the diet, describes them as follows:

Step 1: Low FODMAP: In this phase, the person swaps all high FODMAP foods for low FODMAP options for 2–6 weeks. Some people call this the elimination phase, but Monash stresses that it is a case of substitution rather than elimination.

Step 2: Reintroduction: Under the guidance of a registered dietitian, the person starts reintroducing FODMAP foods into their diet one at a time. This can help identify which foods trigger symptoms. This phase lasts around 6–8 weeks.

Step 3: Personalization: Also known as the maintenance phase, this involves returning to a regular diet as far as possible, limiting only the FODMAP foods that cause IBS symptoms. Eventually, some people may be able to incorporate all or most FODMAPs back into their diet without symptoms.

It is essential to reintroduce foods to see if they cause symptoms, because the aim of the diet is to eliminate only those foods that are troublesome.

Benefits of a low FODMAP diet

Does it work with IBS?

In 2020, some experts concluded that a low FODMAP diet could manage symptoms of IBS. But they insist that people should follow it with caution and only with the guidance of a medical professional.

A 2021 review concludes that the low FODMAP diet can reduce gastrointestinal symptoms and improves quality of life in people with IBS, compared with other diets. Similarly, another 2021 review notes that a low FODMAP diet can help reduce symptoms and improve bowel habits in adults with IBS, and especially those with IBS-D. However, more long-term research on this dietary plan and IBS is still necessary.

While it may show promise, some experts warn that the diet may not be beneficial for everyone with IBS. Possible drawbacks include the following:

• It can be hard to understand, learn, and follow.

• It is a restrictive diet that could increase the risk of disordered eating in some people.

• As a restrictive diet, it could also be hard to follow over time.

• Incorrect use could lead to problems such as nutritional deficiencies and changes to the gut microbiota.

• A lack of standardization of both what the diet involves and food labelling can lead to confusion.

• It may be costly.

• It could worsen some symptoms, such as constipation.

Overall, most researchers seem to agree that, for people with IBS:

• A low FODMAP diet may be beneficial in some cases.

• It is essential to follow the diet with the guidance of a medical professional, as there are some risks.

• More research is necessary to identify the best way to follow the diet and how effective it might be.

Does it help with constipation?

Two symptoms of IBS are constipation and diarrhea.

Some evidence suggests a low FODMAP diet may help reduce constipation in people with IBS, but the picture is likely more complex.

For most people, doctors recommend a high fiber diet to help prevent constipation. Fiber helps food move through the digestive system and encourages the transfer of fluid into the gut, which helps keep stool soft.

Avoiding high FODMAP foods and not replacing them with suitable alternatives could increase the risk of constipation in a person with IBS. Experts recommend working with a dietitian while progressing with the diet to ensure the correct balance and type of fiber to prevent constipation.

A 2021 review notes that a low FODMAP diet may be more helpful for people with IBS where diarrhea is the dominant symptom.

Researchers are still studying how a low FODMAP diet can affect constipation that occurs with IBS.

Does it support weight loss?

Even though following a low FODMAP diet may lead to weight loss in some people, healthcare professionals do not recommend it as a weight loss diet.

Some of the weight loss seen in people following the low FODMAP diet could be due to insufficient calorie intake. This could lead to negative health outcomes, especially if a person has a low weight at the start.

Anyone who is keen to lose weight should speak with their doctor, who will help them find a suitable option.

Foods to avoid and foods to include

Common Foods High in FODMAPs to Avoid

FODMAPs are found in many different foods and beverages. While not an exhaustive list, common foods with high-FODMAP content include:

Fruits:

• Apples

• Pears

• Cherries

- Watermelon

- Peaches

- Plums

- Blackberries

Vegetables:

- Garlic

- Onion

- Leek

- Green onion

- Mushrooms

- Cauliflower

• Snow peas

Grains:

• Wheat

• Rye

Legumes:

• Red kidney beans

• Split peas

• Baked beans

• Falafel

Dairy and milk alternatives:

• Cow's milk

- Yogurt

- Soft cheeses

- Soy milk (made from whole soybeans)

Meat:

- Marinated meats

- Processed meats

Nuts:

- Cashews

- Pistachios

Sweeteners:

- Honey

• High fructose corn syrup

• Sugar alcohols (i.e., sorbitol, xylitol, erythritol)

Some of the most common low FODMAP foods include:

Meat, fish, and meat and fish products without high FODMAP ingredients

Eggs, lactose-free dairy products, hard cheeses, and aged soft cheeses

Certain nuts and seeds, including pine nuts, macadamia nuts, and peanuts

Cantaloupe, grapefruit, honeydew melon, kiwi, citrus fruits, and strawberries

Bell peppers, bok choy, carrots, celery, cucumber, green beans, kale, lettuce, parsnips, potatoes, spinach, squash, sweet potatoes, tomatoes, yams, and zucchini

Corn, oats, quinoa, and rice

Fats, oils, herbs, spices, maple syrup, and stevia

Getting started with the low FODMAP diet

What can you eat on a low FODMAP diet?

Low FODMAP foods include those that do not have certain carbohydrates. This include protein sources, such as chicken, turkey, tofu, and salmon. Other foods include carrot, broccoli, strawberries, oranges, pumpkin seeds, potatoes, and brown rice.

What are the highest FODMAP foods?

The highest FODMAP foods are rich in short-chain carbohydrates. These include foods such as onions, garlic, blackberries, avocados, breaded meats or fish, almonds, and wheat or gluten-based bread.

What happens to your body on low FODMAP diet?

The principle of the FODMAP diet involves identifying if certain foods, known as high FODMAP foods, may trigger symptoms. As these foods may be difficult for some to digest, by determining and limiting them, a person can avoid digestive distress.

What are the negatives of FODMAP diet?

The FODMAP diet may be effective for some, but may not be beneficial for everyone. It is a restrictive diet, and can be difficult to understand and follow. Incorrect use could also lead to health problems. As such, it is advisable to follow the dietary plan under the guidance of a dietitian or medical professional.

Sample Low FODMAP Meal Plans

7-Day Sample Menu

This one-week meal plan was designed for a person who needs about 2,000 calories per day and has no dietary restrictions. Your daily calorie goal may vary. Consider working with a registered dietitian or speaking with a healthcare provider to assess and plan for your dietary needs more accurately.

Each day includes three meals and three Snacks and contains a healthy balance of carbohydrates, fats, and protein. The meal plan also includes fiber, vitamins, minerals, and antioxidants from foods in line with low FODMAP guidelines. You can swap out similar menu items for others, but make sure to use the same cooking method. For example, switching out grilled chicken for grilled fish is fine, but if you fry the fish, then that changes the fat and calories in the meal.

Day 1

Breakfast

• 1 slice sourdough bread

• 1/2 avocado

• 1 fried egg

Macronutrients: 425 calories, 15 grams protein, 42 grams carbohydrates, 23 grams fat

Snack

- 10 almonds

- 1 small orange

Macronutrients: 124 calories, 4 grams protein, 15 grams carbohydrates, 7 grams fat

Lunch

- Chicken Caesar salad wrap with 3 ounces baked chicken breast, 1/2 cup shredded romaine lettuce, 1 tablespoon parmesan cheese, and 2 tablespoons low FODMAP Caesar salad dressing in an 8-inch gluten-free wrap

Macronutrients: 534 calories, 27 grams protein, 30 grams carbohydrates, 33 grams fat

Snack

• 1/2 cup baby carrots

• 1/4 cup garlic-free hummus

Macronutrients: 119 calories, 5 grams protein, 13 grams carbohydrates, 6 grams fat

Dinner

• 4-ounce turkey burger (use ground turkey, and if purchasing a pre-made turkey burger, ensure low-FODMAP-friendly ingredients)

• 1 zucchini sliced into spears, roasted with 1 tbsp olive oil

• 1 regular potato, baked

Macronutrients: 582 calories, 35 grams protein, 40 grams carbohydrates, 33 grams fat

Snack

• 1 cup lactose-free ice cream

Macronutrients: 261 calories, 3 grams protein, 37 grams carbohydrates, 12 grams fat

Daily Totals: 2,045 calories, 89 grams protein, 177 grams carbohydrates, 113 grams fat

Note that beverages are not included in this meal plan. Individual fluid needs vary based on age, sex, activity level, and medical history. For optimal hydration, experts generally recommend drinking approximately 9 cups of water per day for women and 13 cups of water per day for men. When adding beverages to your meal plan, consider their calorie count. Aim to reduce or eliminate consumption of sugar-sweetened beverages, and opt for water when possible.

Day 2

Breakfast

• 1 cup lactose-free yogurt

• 1/4 cup gluten-free granola

• 1/2 cup blueberries

Macronutrients: 298 calories, 16 grams protein, 46 grams carbohydrates, 7 grams fat

Snack

• 2 rice cakes with 1 tablespoon peanut butter

Macronutrients: 164 calories, 5 grams protein, 19 grams carbohydrates, 8 grams fat

Lunch

• 3 ounces tuna mixed with 1/4 avocado on 2 slices of gluten-free bread and a slice of tomato

Macronutrients: 360 calories, 24 grams protein, 34 grams carbohydrates, 14 grams fat

Snack

• 1 ounce cheddar cheese

• 1/2 cup grapes

Macronutrients: 165 calories, 7 grams protein, 15 grams carbohydrates, 9 grams fat

Dinner

• 3 ounces grilled salmon

• 1 cup gluten-free pasta mixed with 1/2 cup low FODMAP tomato sauce (no onions or garlic)

• 1 cup sauteed spinach in 1 tablespoon olive oil

Macronutrients: 669 calories, 31 grams protein, 75 grams carbohydrates, 29 grams fat

Snack

• 2 gluten-free chocolate chip cookies

Macronutrients: 295 calories, 3 grams protein, 39 grams carbohydrates, 15 grams fat

Daily Totals: 1,950 calories, 87 grams protein, 227 grams carbohydrates, 83 grams fat

Day 3

Breakfast

- 1 slice gluten-free bread

- 2 tablespoons peanut butter

- 1 banana

Macronutrients: 393 calories, 10 grams protein, 53 grams carbohydrates, 19 grams fat

Snack

- 1 cup lactose-free yogurt

- 1/2 cup raspberries

Macronutrients: 186 calories, 14 grams protein, 25 grams carbohydrates, 4 grams fat

Lunch

- Vegetable frittata baked with 3 eggs, 1/2 medium sweet potato, 1/2 grated zucchini, and 2 tablespoons parmesan cheese

Macronutrients: 442 calories, 24 grams protein, 17 grams carbohydrates, 31 grams fat

Snack

- 12 corn tortilla chips

- 1/4 cup onion-free guacamole

Macronutrients: 260 calories, 4 grams protein, 30 grams carbohydrates, 16 grams fat

Dinner

- 4 ounces grilled salmon

- 1 cup brown rice, cooked

- 1/2 cup roasted broccoli with 1 tablespoon olive oil

Macronutrients: 599 calories, 31 grams protein, 51 grams carbohydrates, 29 grams fat

Snack

- 1 ounce 70% dark chocolate

• 1 cup plain popcorn

Macronutrients: 214 calories, 3 grams protein, 17 grams carbohydrates, 15 grams fat

Daily Totals: 2,094 calories, 85 grams protein, 193 carbohydrates, 114 grams fat

Day 4

Breakfast

• 1/2 cup cooked oatmeal in water

• 1 tablespoon peanut butter

• 1/2 cup blueberries

Macronutrients: 302 calories, 10 grams protein, 43 grams carbohydrates, 12 grams fat

Snack

- 1 cup cubed cantaloupe

- 10 almonds

Macronutrients: 132 calories, 4 grams protein, 16 grams carbohydrates, 7 grams fat

Lunch

- 4 ounces sliced turkey, 1/2 avocado, 1/2 cup spinach, and 2 slices tomato in an 8-inch gluten-free wrap

Macronutrients: 475 calories, 25 grams protein, 50 grams carbohydrates, 22 grams fat

Snack

- 10 2-inch long gluten-free pretzels twists

- 1/4 cup garlic-free hummus

Macronutrients: 330 calories, 11 grams protein, 57 grams carbohydrates, 8 grams fat

Dinner

- 4 ounces cubed tofu, 1/2 cup broccoli, 1/2 chopped red bell pepper stir-fried in one tablespoon olive oil

- 2 tablespoons garlic-free teriyaki sauce

- 1 cup rice noodles

Macronutrients: 479 calories, 19 grams protein, 59 grams carbohydrates, 20 grams fat

Snack

- 5 large strawberries

- 2 tablespoons almond butter

Macronutrients: 225 calories, 7 grams protein, 13 grams carbohydrates, 18 grams fat

Daily Totals: 1,943 calories, 76 grams protein, 236 grams carbohydrates, 87 grams fat

Day 5

Breakfast

- 1 slice sourdough bread

- 1/2 avocado

- 1 fried egg

Macronutrients: 345 calories, 14 grams protein, 38 grams carbohydrates, 16 grams fat

Snack

- 10 walnuts

- 1/4 cup dried cranberries

Macronutrients: 256 calories, 3 grams protein, 36 grams carbohydrates, 14 grams fat

Lunch

- Hummus wrap with 1/4 cup garlic-free hummus, lettuce, tomatoes, cucumber, 1/4 cup olives, and 1/4 cup feta cheese on an 8-inch gluten-free wrap

Macronutrients: 435 calories, 17 grams protein, 48 grams carbohydrates, 21 grams fat

Snack

• 2 cups plain salted popcorn

Macronutrients: 88 calories, 1 grams protein, 9 grams carbohydrates, 5 grams fat

Dinner

• 3 ounces grilled steak

• 1 cup cooked brown rice

• 1 zucchini cut into spears and roasted in 1 tablespoon olive oil

Macronutrients: 594 calories, 28 grams protein, 49 grams carbohydrates, 31 grams fat

Snack

• 1/4 cup dark chocolate chips

Macronutrients: 202 calories, 2 grams protein, 27 grams carbohydrates, 13 grams fat

Daily Totals: 1,918 calories, 65 grams protein, 206 grams carbohydrates, 100 grams fat

Day 6

Breakfast

• 4-inch gluten-free bagel

• 2 tablespoons cream cheese

- 1 ounce smoked salmon

Macronutrients: 412 calories, 18 grams protein, 57 grams carbohydrates, 13 grams fat

Snack

- 1 small banana

- 1 tablespoon peanut butter

Macronutrients: 184 calories, 5 grams protein, 27 grams carbohydrates, 8 grams fat

Lunch

- 2 slices gluten-free bread

- 1/2 avocado

- 2 poached eggs

Macronutrients: 471 calories, 18 grams protein, 38 grams carbohydrates, 29 grams fat

Snack

- 1/2 cup baby carrots

- 1/4 cup garlic-free hummus

Macronutrients: 119 calories, 5 grams protein, 13 grams carbohydrates, 6 grams fat

Dinner

- 1 1/2 cups rice pasta with 1/2 cup garlic and onion-free tomato sauce, 1 cup cubed eggplant chopped and sauteed in 1 tablespoon olive oil, and 2 tablespoons parmesan cheese

Macronutrients: 497 calories, 12 grams protein, 80 grams carbohydrates, 20 grams fat

Snack

• 1 cup lactose-free ice cream

Macronutrients: 273 calories, 5 grams protein, 31 grams carbohydrates, 15 grams fat

Daily Totals: 1,955 calories, 62 grams protein, 246 grams carbohydrates, 90 grams fat

Day 7

Breakfast

• 3/4 cup coconut yogurt

• 1/4 cup gluten-free granola

- 1/2 cup blueberries

Macronutrients: 318 calories, 11 grams protein, 63 grams carbohydrates, 3 grams fat

Snack

- 2 rice cakes

- 2 tbsp almond butter

Macronutrients: 266 calories, 8 grams protein, 21 grams carbohydrates, 18 grams fat

Lunch

- 4 ounces sliced turkey

- 1 tablespoon whole grain mustard, 1 slice of tomato, and lettuce leaf

- 2 slices of gluten-free bread

- 10 baby carrots

Macronutrients: 335 calories, 20 grams protein, 45 grams carbohydrates, 9 grams fat

Snack

- 1 medium tangerine

- 10 walnut halves

Macronutrients: 179 calories, 4 grams protein, 15 grams carbohydrates, 14 grams fat

Dinner

- 4 ounces grilled salmon

- 1 cup cooked quinoa

- 1/2 cup steamed green beans

Macronutrients: 477 calories, 34 grams protein, 44 grams carbohydrates, 18 grams fat

Snack

- 2 ounces 70% dark chocolate

- 1/2 cup raspberries

Macronutrients: 371 calories, 5 grams protein, 33 grams carbohydrates, 25 grams fat

Daily Totals: 1,947 calories, 83 grams protein, 222 grams carbohydrates, 86 grams fat

Tips for Shopping and Meal Preparation

Shopping for a low-FODMAP diet can be expensive. There are ways, though, to make sure your grocery bill doesn't break the bank:

1. Plan your meals and write a shopping list

Planning out your weekly meals means you can write a detailed shopping list. This helps you from wandering aimlessly around the supermarket and should also help stop impulse buying!

2. Check out independent greengrocers, Asian supermarkets, and butchers in your area

They often have lower prices and good-quality produce. Independent butchers generally allow you to buy the exact quantity of meat you need, which can save you a lot of money.

3. Cook extra for dinner and take leftovers for lunch

It's much cheaper to cook in bulk, and it reduces the amount of meal prep work you need to do each week. Leftovers can be stored in containers and taken to work the next day or popped in the freezer for a later date.

4. Re-grow your spring onions and leeks

A low-FODMAP diet means we can only use the green tips of both spring onions and leeks. Once you have harvested the tips, place the spring onion bulbs and leek bulbs in glasses of water on your window sill. They will begin to reshoot after a couple of days. After about a week transfer them into a planter box and then continue to harvest the green tips as you need them.

5. Use frozen vegetables (especially green beans) and berries

These are just as nutritious as fresh, and generally much cheaper. Using frozen produce also reduces waste as it keeps for months in the freezer.

6. Invest in a selection of dried herbs or grow your own fresh herbs

Dried herbs are relatively cheap compared to fresh herbs and they last for months in the pantry. If using dry instead of fresh, reduce the amount by three. This means if a recipe calls for one tablespoon of fresh herbs, use just one teaspoon of dried herbs (1 tablespoon = 3 teaspoons). Another cost-saving tip is to grow your favourite herbs in pots on your deck or windowsill. Preferred herbs to grow are parsley, basil, coriander and chives.

7. Focus on using potatoes, rice, and rice noodles as fillers in your meals

Keep gluten-free pasta as an occasional treat. Unwashed potatoes are cheaper than washed potatoes. Also, the trick to good rice noodles is to avoid overcooking them, so check the noodles two minutes before they are meant to be ready.

8. Save money on meat

Tinned fish like tuna and salmon, lean minced meat and eggs are cheap and versatile sources of protein. When choosing tinned fish make sure you buy plain flavours and check for high-FODMAP ingredients. Remember to bulk out your meat-based meals with several low-FODMAP vegetables and low-FODMAP fillers like rice or potato.

9. Make your own lactose-free milk

Lactose-free milk is significantly more expensive than standard cow's milk, but you can make your own by adding lactase drops to standard cow's milk and leaving it for 24 hours before consuming. The lactase enzymes digest the lactose, making it low FODMAP. Lactase drops are available over the counter at most pharmacies.

10. Do your own gluten-free baking

Gluten-free baking from the supermarket is expensive. Try baking your own gluten-free items and storing them in the freezer. That way you always have a low-FODMAP treat when you need one. For low-FODMAP baking ideas check out www.alittlebityummy.com.

11. Carry a water bottle

Key to having a healthy body is staying hydrated. Bottled water is expensive and the plastic waste we generate each day from disposable bottles is a threat to the environment. So do your budget and the environment a favour and carry a reusable water bottle!

Common Challenges and How to Overcome Them

Fast food and restaurant food are often high in FODMAPs, which can make dining out difficult when you're following a low FODMAP meal plan. Still, that doesn't mean that you can't find low FODMAP foods when you're dining out.

Before you leave the house, consider looking at menu options ahead of time. By checking the menu before you go, you'll be able to familiarize yourself with some of the low FODMAP food choices available to you.

Once you're at the restaurant or establishment, don't hesitate to ask questions about the menu options. Let the server know that you have dietary concerns and will need to avoid some things. Sometimes, you may even be able to make adjustments, like asking for dressing on the side or exchanging a high FODMAP ingredient for a lower FODMAP one.

You may want to look for restaurants that offer plenty of gluten- and dairy-free options or those that can make food allergen-safe.

CHAPTER 2
INCORPORATING HIGH FIBER FOODS

Fiber feeds "good" gut bacteria

The bacteria that live in the human body outnumber the body's cells 10 to 1. Bacteria live on the skin, in the mouth, and in the nose, but the great majority live in the gut, primarily the large intestine.

Five hundred to 1,000 different species of bacteria live in the intestine, totaling about 38 trillion cells. These gut bacteria are also known as the gut flora.

This is not a bad thing. In fact, there is a mutually beneficial relationship between you and some of the bacteria that live in your digestive system.

You provide food, shelter, and a safe habitat for the bacteria. In return, they take care of some things that the human body cannot do on its own.

Of the many different kinds of bacteria, some are crucial for various aspects of your health, including weight, blood sugar control, immune function, and even brain function.

You may wonder what this has to do with fiber. Just like any other organism, bacteria need to eat to get energy to survive and function.

The problem is that most carbs, proteins, and fats are absorbed into the bloodstream before they make it to the large intestine, leaving little for the gut flora.

This is where fiber comes in. Human cells don't have the enzymes to digest fiber, so it reaches the large intestine relatively unchanged.

However, intestinal bacteria do have the enzymes to digest many of these fibers.

This is the most important reason that (some) dietary fibers are essential for health. They feed the "good" bacteria in the intestine, functioning as prebiotics.

In this way, they promote the growth of "good" gut bacteria, which can have various positive effects on health.

The friendly bacteria produce nutrients for the body, including short-chain fatty acids such as acetate, propionate, and butyrate, of which butyrate appears to be the most important.

These short-chain fatty acids can feed the cells in the colon, leading to reduced gut inflammation and improvements in digestive disorders such as irritable bowel syndrome, Crohn's disease, and ulcerative colitis.

When the bacteria ferment the fiber, they also produce gases. This is why high fiber diets can cause flatulence and stomach discomfort in some people. These side effects usually go away with time as your body adjusts.

Lower Odds of Heart Disease

According to a 2022 BMC Public Health study, a higher fiber intake was associated with a reduced risk for cardiovascular disease (CVD) in a large group of Americans. Researchers don't completely understand how fiber works, but they think that soluble fiber plays a role in decreasing lipid uptake from the intestinal tract, resulting in lower blood levels of cholesterol according to a 2023 Advances in Nutrition review. In addition, experts say that dietary fiber reduces inflammation which can result in CVD in a 2022 JAMA Network Open article.

Some types of fiber can help you lose weight

Certain types of fiber can help you lose weight by reducing your appetite.

In fact, some studies show that increasing dietary fiber can cause weight loss by automatically reducing calorie intake.

Fiber can soak up water in the intestine, slowing the absorption of nutrients and increasing feelings of fullness.

However, this depends on the type of fiber. Some types have no effect on weight, while certain soluble fibers can have a significant effect.

A good example of an effective fiber supplement for weight loss is glucomannan.

Fiber can reduce blood sugar spikes after a high carb meal

High fiber foods tend to have a lower glycemic index than refined carb sources, which have been stripped of most of their fiber.

However, scientists believe that only high viscosity, soluble fibers have this property.

Including these viscous, soluble fibers in your carb-containing meals may cause smaller spikes in blood sugar.

This is important, especially if you're following a high carb diet. In this case, the fiber can reduce the likelihood of the carbs raising your blood sugar to harmful levels.

That said, if you have blood sugar issues, you should consider reducing your carb intake — especially your intake of low fiber, refined carbs such as white flour and added sugar.

Fiber can reduce cholesterol, but the effect isn't huge

Viscous, soluble fiber can also reduce your cholesterol levels.

However, the effect isn't nearly as impressive as you might expect.

A review of 67 controlled studies found that consuming 2–10 grams of soluble fiber per day reduced total cholesterol by only 1.7 mg/dl and LDL (bad) cholesterol by 2.2 mg/dl, on average.

But this also depends on the viscosity of the fiber. Some studies have found impressive reductions in cholesterol with increased fiber intake.

Whether this has any meaningful effects in the long term is unknown, although many observational studies show that people who eat more fiber have a lower risk of heart disease.

Fiber might reduce the risk of colorectal cancer

Colorectal cancer is the third leading cause of cancer deaths in the world.

Many studies have linked a high intake of fiber-rich foods with a reduced risk of colon cancer.

However, whole, high fiber foods like fruits, vegetables, and whole grains contain various other healthy nutrients and antioxidants that may affect cancer risk.

Therefore, it's difficult to isolate the effects of fiber from other factors in healthy, whole-food diets. To date, no strong evidence proves that fiber has cancer-preventive effects.

Yet, since fiber may help keep the colon wall healthy, many scientists believe that fiber plays an important role.

More Regular Bowel Movements

One of the main benefits of increasing fiber intake is reduced constipation.

Fiber is believed to help absorb water, increase the bulk of stool, and speed up the movement of stool through the intestine. However, the evidence is fairly conflicting.

Longer Life

A 2022 review in the Journal of Translational Medicine found that people who ate enough total fiber—which includes soluble and insoluble fibers—had a lower chance of dying early from anything, including cardiovascular disease and cancer. This means that even if you were to get heart disease, cancer or another condition, consuming enough fiber may protect you from dying from it.

Some studies show that increasing fiber can improve symptoms of constipation, but other studies show that removing fiber improves constipation. The effects depend on the type of fiber.

In one study in 63 individuals with chronic constipation, going on a low fiber diet fixed their problem. The individuals who remained on a high fiber diet saw no improvement.

In general, fiber that increases the water content of your stool has a laxative effect, while fiber that adds to the dry mass of stool without increasing its water content may have a constipating effect.

Soluble fibers that form a gel in the digestive tract and are not fermented by gut bacteria are often effective. A good example of a gel-forming fiber is psyllium.

Other types of fiber, such as sorbitol, have a laxative effect by drawing water into the colon. Prunes are a good source of sorbitol.

Choosing the right type of fiber may help your constipation, but taking the wrong supplements can do the opposite.

For this reason, you should consult a healthcare professional before taking fiber supplements for constipation.

All-Natural Detox

Fiber naturally scrubs and promotes the elimination of toxins from your GI tract. Soluble fiber soaks up potentially harmful compounds, such as excess estrogen and unhealthy fats, before they can be absorbed by the body. And because insoluble fiber makes things move along more quickly, it limits the amount of time that chemicals like BPA, mercury and pesticides stay in your system. The faster they go through you, the less chance they have to cause harm.

Strong Bones

Some types of soluble fiber — known as prebiotics — have been shown to contribute to a greater bioavailability of minerals, like calcium, in your colon. The increase in bioavailability supports maintain bone density, according to a 2018 review in the journal Calcified Tissue International. Prebiotics provide food for your beneficial gut bacteria and can be found in certain fruits, vegetables, nuts and whole grains, such as asparagus, bananas, walnuts, onions, legumes, wheat and oats.

High fiber foods that are low in FODMAPs

Fruits and Vegetables

Blueberries 1 cup blueberries contains 4 grams of fiber

Carrots 1 cup sliced raw carrot contains 3 grams of fiber

Chard ½ cup cooked chard contains 2 grams of fiber

Collards ½ cup cooked collards contain 4 grams of fiber (collards contain osmotic sugars that might loosen BMs)

Eggplant 1 cup cubed raw eggplant contains 2.5 grams of fiber

Kale 2 cups raw kale contains 3.5 grams of fiber

Kiwi 2 small kiwis contain 4 grams of fiber

Oranges 1 medium orange contains 3 grams of fiber

Parsnip 1 medium parsnip contains 3 grams of fiber

Potato with Skin 1 medium potato with skin contains 4 grams of fiber

Raspberry ⅓ cup (58g) raspberries contains 3 grams of fiber

Low FODMAP Whole Grains

Brown Rice 1 cup cooked brown rice contains 3 grams of fiber

Oats ½ cup dry rolled oats contains 5.5 grams of fiber

Popcorn 4 cups air-popped popcorn contains 5 grams of fiber

Quinoa 1 cup cooked quinoa contains 5.5 grams of fiber

Nuts and Seeds

Chia seeds 2 tablespoons whole chia seeds contain 7 grams of fiber

Flax 1 tablespoon ground flax contains 2 grams of fiber

Peanuts 32 peanuts (1 ounce) contains 2.5 grams of fiber

Walnuts 10 walnut halves contains 2 grams of fiber

Legumes

Chickpeas ¼ cup canned, rinsed chickpeas contains 2 grams of fiber

Edamame ½ cup cooked shelled edamame contains 4 grams of fiber

Lentils ¼ cup canned, rinsed lentils contains 2 grams of fiber

Tofu 1 cup tofu contains 2.5 grams of fiber

Tempeh ½ cup of tempeh contains 6 grams of fiber

How to increase fiber intake gradually

Below are tips for fitting in more fiber:

Jump-start your day

For breakfast choose a high-fiber breakfast cereal — 5 or more grams of fiber a serving. Opt for cereals with "whole grain," "bran" or "fiber" in the name. Or add a few tablespoons of unprocessed wheat bran to your favorite cereal.

Switch to whole grains

Consume at least half of all grains as whole grains. Look for breads that list whole wheat, whole-wheat flour or another whole grain as the first ingredient on the label and have at least 2 grams of dietary fiber a serving. Experiment with brown rice, wild rice, barley, whole-wheat pasta and bulgur wheat.

Bulk up baked goods

Substitute whole-grain flour for half or all of the white flour when baking. Try adding crushed bran cereal, unprocessed wheat bran or uncooked oatmeal to muffins, cakes and cookies.

Lean on legumes

Beans, peas and lentils are excellent sources of fiber. Add kidney beans to canned soup or a green salad. Or make nachos with refried black beans, lots of fresh veggies, whole-wheat tortilla chips and salsa.

Eat more fruit and vegetables

Fruits and vegetables are rich in fiber, as well as vitamins and minerals. Try to eat five or more servings daily.

Make snacks count

Fresh fruits, raw vegetables, low-fat popcorn and whole-grain crackers are all good choices. A handful of nuts or dried fruits also is a healthy, high-fiber snack — although be aware that nuts and dried fruits are high in calories.

High-fiber foods are good for your health. But adding too much fiber too quickly can promote intestinal gas, abdominal bloating and cramping. Increase fiber in your diet gradually over a few weeks. This allows the natural bacteria in your digestive system to adjust to the change.

Also, drink plenty of water. Fiber works best when it absorbs water, making your stool soft and bulky.

Tips for Shopping and Meal Preparation

Shopping for a low-FODMAP diet can be expensive. There are ways, though, to make sure your grocery bill doesn't break the bank:

1. Plan your meals and write a shopping list

Planning out your weekly meals means you can write a detailed shopping list. This helps you from wandering aimlessly around the supermarket and should also help stop impulse buying!

2. Check out independent greengrocers, Asian supermarkets, and butchers in your area

They often have lower prices and good-quality produce. Independent butchers generally allow you to buy the exact quantity of meat you need, which can save you a lot of money.

3. Cook extra for dinner and take leftovers for lunch

It's much cheaper to cook in bulk, and it reduces the amount of meal prep work you need to do each week. Leftovers can be stored in containers and taken to work the next day or popped in the freezer for a later date.

4. Re-grow your spring onions and leeks

A low-FODMAP diet means we can only use the green tips of both spring onions and leeks. Once you have harvested the tips, place the spring onion bulbs and leek bulbs in glasses of water on your window sill. They will begin to reshoot after a couple of days. After about a week transfer them into a planter box and then continue to harvest the green tips as you need them.

5. Use frozen vegetables (especially green beans) and berries

These are just as nutritious as fresh, and generally much cheaper. Using frozen produce also reduces waste as it keeps for months in the freezer.

6. Invest in a selection of dried herbs or grow your own fresh herbs

Dried herbs are relatively cheap compared to fresh herbs and they last for months in the pantry. If using dry instead of fresh, reduce the amount by three. This means if a recipe calls for one tablespoon of fresh herbs, use just one teaspoon of dried herbs (1 tablespoon = 3 teaspoons). Another cost-saving tip is to grow your favourite herbs in pots on your deck or windowsill. Preferred herbs to grow are parsley, basil, coriander and chives.

7. Focus on using potatoes, rice, and rice noodles as fillers in your meals

Keep gluten-free pasta as an occasional treat. Unwashed potatoes are cheaper than washed potatoes. Also, the trick to good rice noodles is to avoid overcooking them, so check the noodles two minutes before they are meant to be ready.

8. Save money on meat

Tinned fish like tuna and salmon, lean minced meat and eggs are cheap and versatile sources of protein. When choosing tinned fish make sure you buy plain flavours and check for high-FODMAP ingredients. Remember to bulk out your meat-based meals with several low-FODMAP vegetables and low-FODMAP fillers like rice or potato.

9. Make your own lactose-free milk

Lactose-free milk is significantly more expensive than standard cow's milk, but you can make your own by adding lactase drops to standard cow's milk and leaving it for 24 hours before consuming. The lactase enzymes digest the lactose, making it low FODMAP. Lactase drops are available over the counter at most pharmacies.

10. Do your own gluten-free baking

Gluten-free baking from the supermarket is expensive. Try baking your own gluten-free items and storing them in the freezer. That way you always have a low-FODMAP treat when you need one. For low-FODMAP baking ideas check out www.alittlebityummy.com.

11. Carry a water bottle

Key to having a healthy body is staying hydrated. Bottled water is expensive and the plastic waste we generate each day from disposable bottles is a threat to the environment. So do your budget and the environment a favour and carry a reusable water bottle.

CHAPTER 3
THE GLUTEN-FREE APPROACH

Gluten is a family of proteins found in wheat, barley, rye, and spelt. Its name comes from the Latin word for glue. It gives flour a sticky consistency when it's mixed with water.

This glue-like property helps gluten create a sticky network that gives bread the ability to rise when baked. It also gives bread a chewy and satisfying texture.

Some people have uncomfortable gastrointestinal symptoms after eating foods that contain gluten. Severe reactions can occur in people diagnosed with celiac disease.

Celiac disease is an autoimmune disorder in which the body mistakenly attacks itself after exposure to gluten. Celiac disease affects at least 1% of the population in the Western world and can damage the intestines.

If eating gluten makes you feel uncomfortable, a doctor may recommend screening for celiac disease.

But many people go gluten-free despite not having celiac disease or other similar health conditions that necessitate eliminating gluten. People who follow a gluten-free diet for nonmedical reasons may be seeking weight loss, better focus, increased energy, or a less-bloated belly, all potential benefits touted commonly by wellness influencers.

There's no question that the gluten-free diet has become popular for nonmedical reasons. Indeed, the number of people on the gluten-free diet who do not have celiac disease is almost double the number of people diagnosed with celiac disease. Research shows about 2.7 million people in the United States follow a gluten-free diet without having celiac. The demand for gluten-free foods in the United States is also significant, with sales of gluten-free products totaling more than $15.5 billion in 2016.

 That number is expected to reach more than $17 billion by 2027.

How does the Gluten-Free Diet work?

Eat nutrient-rich grains, including rice, millet, quinoa and amaranth.

You'll want to steer clear of wheat, barley, rye and triticale, a hybrid grain produced by crossing rye and wheat. Wheat may be called by other names; varieties of the grain include bulgur, semolina, spelt and farro.

Choose whole, unprocessed foods. Plain meat, poultry, fish, fruits, vegetables, nuts, beans, legumes, eggs and dairy are all gluten-free. Beware of seasonings and marinades, which often contain gluten.

Beware of the bevy of gluten-free processed foods that may fill you with empty calories. These products often compensate for gluten with extra sugar and fat. Plus, these products routinely swap whole-wheat flours, which provide nutrients, with less-nutritious, high-glycemic alternatives.

Benefits of a gluten-free diet

May help relieve digestive symptoms

Most people try a gluten-free diet to help treat digestive problems. This includes many symptoms like:

- bloating

- diarrhea or constipation

- gas

- fatigue

Research shows that following a gluten-free diet can help ease digestive symptoms for people with celiac disease and NCGS.

According to one study involving 856 people with celiac disease, those who did not follow a gluten-free diet experienced significantly more diarrhea, indigestion, and stomach pain compared with those on a gluten-free diet.

Can help reduce chronic inflammation in those with celiac disease

Inflammation is a natural process that helps the body treat and heal infection.

Sometimes inflammation can get out of hand and last weeks, months, or even years. This is known as chronic inflammation and may lead to various health problems in the long run.

A gluten-free diet can help reduce chronic inflammation in those with celiac disease.

In fact, a gluten-free diet can help reduce markers of inflammation, like antibody levels, and may also help treat gut damage that gluten-related inflammation in those with celiac disease causes.

People with NCGS may also have low levels of inflammation, but it's not completely clear if a gluten-free diet can help reduce their inflammation.

May help boost energy

People with celiac disease often feel tired or sluggish. They may also experience brain fog, which is characterized by confusion, forgetfulness, and difficulty focusing.

These symptoms may result from nutrient deficiencies caused by damage to the gut. For example, an iron deficiency can lead to anemia, which is common in celiac disease.

If you have celiac disease, switching to a gluten-free diet may help boost your energy levels and relieve tiredness and sluggishness.

According to one literature review, people with celiac disease experienced significantly more fatigue than those without celiac disease. Additionally, five of the seven studies included in the review concluded that following a gluten-free diet was effective at reducing fatigue.

Possible weight changes

You may experience some weight loss when you first start following a gluten-free diet.

Some weight loss may be due to eliminating many processed foods like cookies, cakes, and other snack foods. But some weight loss may occur due to the restrictive nature of the diet or the lack of planned balanced meals.

Gluten-free options do not always mean they are "healthy" or "nutritious." Some processed gluten-free products like cakes, pastries, and snacks can be high in calories with few nutrients. They can cause weight gain if they're eaten regularly.

A gluten-free diet is not considered a weight loss diet. It's important that everyone focus on eating more fruits, vegetables, lean proteins, dairy, and healthy fats in place of more highly processed foods.

Other benefits of following a gluten-free diet includes:

• **Irritable Bowel Syndrome:** One study of 140 IBS patients found that following a gluten-free diet for 12 weeks led to significant improvement of gastrointestinal symptoms.

• **Schizophrenia:** A research review of nine studies found that six of them demonstrated beneficial effects of a gluten-free diet for people with schizophrenia, including improved functioning and decreased symptoms severity.

• **Fibromyalgia:** One small study of 20 women with fibromyalgia and gluten sensitivity found that all of the study participants reported improved symptoms while following a gluten-free diet. Fifteen of the women experienced dramatic improvement in chronic widespread pain, indicating remission from their disease.

• **Endometriosis**: A study of 207 women with endometriosis found 75 percent reported a significant change in painful symptoms after following a gluten-free diet for 12 months.

Gluten-free grains and their nutritional benefits

1. Sorghum

Sorghum is typically cultivated as both a cereal grain and animal feed. It's also used to produce sorghum syrup, a type of sweetener, as well as some alcoholic beverages.

This gluten-free grain contains beneficial plant compounds that act as antioxidants to reduce oxidative stress and lower your risk of chronic disease.

Additionally, sorghum is rich in fiber and can help slow the absorption of sugar to keep your blood sugar levels steady.

One study compared blood sugar and insulin levels in 10 people after eating a muffin made with either sorghum or whole-wheat flour. The sorghum muffin led to a greater reduction in both blood sugar and insulin than the whole-wheat muffin.

A 2010 test-tube and animal study suggests that black sorghum bran possesses significant anti-inflammatory properties due to its high content of these plant compounds.

One cup (192 grams) of sorghum contains 13 grams of fiber, 20 grams of protein, and 19% of the daily value for iron.

Sorghum has a mild flavor and can be ground into flour for baking gluten-free goods. It can also replace barley in recipes like mushroom-barley soup.

2. Quinoa

Quinoa has quickly become one of the most popular gluten-free grains. It's incredibly versatile and a good source of fiber and plant-based protein.

It's also one of the healthiest grains, boasting a high amount of antioxidants that may help reduce your risk of disease.

Additionally, quinoa is a good source of protein and one of the few plant foods considered a complete protein source.

While most plant foods are lacking in one or two of the essential amino acids required by your body, quinoa contains all eight. This makes it an excellent plant-based source of protein.

One cup (185 grams) of cooked quinoa provides 8 grams of protein and 5 grams of fiber. It's also packed with micronutrients and fulfills much of your daily magnesium, manganese, and phosphorus requirements.

Quinoa is the perfect ingredient to make gluten-free crusts and casseroles. Quinoa flour can also be used to make pancakes, tortillas, or quick bread.

3. Oats

Oats are very healthy. They also stand out as one of the best sources of oat beta-glucan, a type of soluble fiber with advantages for your health.

A review of 28 studies found that beta-glucan decreased both LDL (bad) and total cholesterol without affecting HDL (good) cholesterol.

Other studies have shown that beta-glucan may slow the absorption of sugar and lower blood sugar and insulin levels.

One cup (81 grams) of dry oats provides 8 grams of fiber and 11 grams of protein. It is also high in magnesium, zinc, selenium, and thiamine (vitamin B1).

Although oats are naturally gluten-free, many brands of oats may contain trace amounts of gluten. Oat products may become contaminated with gluten when they are harvested and processed.

If you have celiac disease or a gluten sensitivity, be sure to look for oats labeled as certified gluten-free.

Keep in mind that a small proportion of people with celiac disease may be sensitive to avenin, a protein found in oats. However, oats that are gluten-free should be fine for the majority of gluten-intolerant people.

A hot bowl of oatmeal is the most popular way to enjoy oats, but you can also add oats to pancakes, granola bars, or parfaits for extra fiber and nutrients.

4. Buckwheat

Despite its name, buckwheat is a grain-like seed that's unrelated to wheat and gluten-free.

It provides plenty of antioxidants, including high amounts of two specific types — rutin and quercetin.

Some animal studies have suggested that rutin may help improve symptoms of Alzheimer's disease. Meanwhile, quercetin has been shown to lower inflammation and oxidative stress.

Eating buckwheat may also help reduce some risk factors for heart disease.

In one study, buckwheat intake was associated with lower total and LDL (bad) cholesterol, as well as a higher ratio of HDL (good) to total cholesterol.

Another study observed similar findings, showing that those who ate buckwheat had a lower risk of high blood pressure, high cholesterol, and high blood sugar.

One cup (168 grams) of cooked buckwheat groats delivers 5 grams of fiber and 6 grams of protein and is a rich source of magnesium, copper, and manganese.

Try soba noodles made from buckwheat as a gluten-free swap for traditional pasta. Alternatively, use buckwheat to add a bit of crunch to soups, salads, or even veggie burgers.

5. Amaranth

Amaranth has a rich history as one of the staple foods for the Inca, Maya, and Aztec civilizations.

Moreover, it is a highly nutritious grain with some impressive health benefits.

A 2014 test-tube study suggests that the compounds in amaranth block inflammation by preventing the activation of a pathway that triggers inflammation.

Thanks to its high fiber content, amaranth may also decrease several heart disease risk factors.

In fact, one animal study found that amaranth seeds decreased both blood triglycerides and LDL (bad) cholesterol levels.

One cup (246 grams) of cooked amaranth contains 5 grams of fiber and 9 grams of protein. It also meets 29% of your daily iron needs and contains a good amount of magnesium, phosphorus, and manganese.

You can use amaranth as a substitute for other grains, such as rice or couscous. Amaranth that has been cooked and then chilled can also be used in place of cornstarch as a thickening agent for soups, jellies, or sauces.

6. Teff

As one of the smallest grains in the world, teff is a tiny but powerful grain.

Despite being just 1/100 the size of a kernel of wheat, teff packs a nutritional punch.

Teff is high in protein, which can help promote satiety, reduce cravings, and boost metabolism.

It also fulfills a good portion of your daily fiber needs. Fiber is an important part of the diet and is associated with weight loss, reduced appetite, and improved regularity.

One cup (252 grams) of cooked teff contains 10 grams of protein and 7 grams of fiber. It also provides plenty of B vitamins, especially thiamine.

For gluten-free baking, try substituting teff in part or in whole for wheat flour. Teff can also be mixed into chili, made into porridge, or used as a natural way to thicken dishes.

7. Corn

Corn, or maize, is among the most popular gluten-free cereal grains consumed around the world.

In addition to being high in fiber, corn is a rich source of the carotenoids lutein and zeaxanthin, which are plant pigments that act as antioxidants.

Studies show that lutein and zeaxanthin can benefit eye health by decreasing the risk of cataracts and age-related macular degeneration, two common causes of vision loss in older adults.

One study found that those with a high intake of carotenoids had a 43% lower risk of age-related macular degeneration compared with those with a low intake.

One cup (149 grams) of sweet corn contains 4 grams of fiber and 5 grams of protein. It's also high in pantothenic acid and a good source of vitamin B6, thiamine, and manganese.

Corn can be boiled, grilled, or roasted for a healthy side dish to a well-balanced meal. Enjoy it right off the cob or add it to a salad, soup, or casserole.

8. Brown rice

Although brown and white rice come from the same grain, white rice has had the bran and germ of the grain removed during processing.

Thus, brown rice has more fiber and a higher amount of many micronutrients, making it one of the healthiest gluten-free grains around.

Both varieties of rice are gluten-free, but studies show that replacing white rice with brown rice comes with added health benefits.

In fact, choosing brown rice in place of white rice can lead to decreased risks of diabetes, weight gain, and heart disease.

One cup (202 grams) of cooked brown rice contains 3 grams of fiber and 6 grams of protein. It also provides a good portion of your magnesium and selenium needs for the day.

Brown rice makes a delicious side dish on its own or can be combined with vegetables and a lean source of protein to create a filling meal.

How to avoid hidden sources of gluten

The following tips can help you prevent cross-contamination in your own food preparations at home and avoid gluten-containing food when you eat out:

Store gluten-free and gluten-containing foods in different places.

Keep cooking surfaces and food storage areas clean.

Wash dishes and cooking equipment thoroughly.

Toast bread in the oven — or consider separate toasters — to avoid cross-contamination.

Read restaurant menus online ahead of time if possible to be sure there are options for you.

Eat out early or late when a restaurant is less busy and better able to address your needs.

Gluten-free baking and cooking tips

Baking Times

Baking times can vary depending on the type of pan you use. Make sure to check the manufacturer's advice of the pan you're using and use the pan that for which your particular recipe is calling. Oven temperatures can also vary from kitchen to kitchen, so it is important to tune or test.

Essential to this is purchasing an oven thermometer and adjusting the temperature accordingly. Lastly, placing your baked goods in the center of a pre-heated oven will help with even baking. Remember, baking times for gluten-free foods vary greatly, and it's important to keep a constant eye on your creation to monitor for the colors and textures that indicate doneness. These recipes often call for longer baking times at a lower temperature compared to traditional recipes.

Flavor

New bakers should try adding extra vanilla and/or spices to recipes. Gluten-free flours often have unique tastes, and adding additional flavoring to recipes will help cover up these unfamiliar flavors.

Freshness

Gluten-free grains and starches have a shelf-life, so it's recommended to buy them in smaller quantities and store in the refrigerator or freezer to prolong the essential properties of your ingredients. Some flours can even be made at home buy purchasing the whole grain and then processing with a coffee grinder.

To avoid baked goods becoming soggy, transfer to a wire rack as soon as possible after baking to ensure that they cool properly. Left-overs can then be frozen to preserve freshness, just make sure to thaw them completely before eating.

Leavening & High Altitude

2 teaspoons of baking powder per cup of gluten-free flour is necessary to ensure proper leavening.

Baking soda and buttermilk can be used to leaven instead of baking powder, but 1-1/8 teaspoon of cream of tartar should be added for each 1/2 teaspoon baking soda used. Dissolving leaveners in liquid prior to adding to dough will give a better rise to the product.

Gluten-free baking at high altitude requires less liquid and either a higher oven temperature or a longer baking time. Start with omitting 2 tablespoons of liquid and increasing the oven temperature by 25° F.

Moisture

There are many ways to increase moisture in a recipe. In general, recipes that call for pureed fruit, sour cream or yogurt are ones you can rely on for a moist product. In case your recipe does not call for these things, using brown sugar instead of white sugar to add moisture. Honey and agave as a sugar substitute can enhance moisture as well, but be aware that you should cut down slightly on the other liquids you are using in the recipe, as honey and agave are not solid ingredients. Adding an extra egg or oil can also help, but use caution.

Nutrition

Substituting 1/4 cup ground flaxseed in 1/4 cup water for 1/4 cup flour will increase nutrition in any recipe.

Structure

As you probably know, gluten is the ingredient most responsible for the structure of baked goods in traditional recipes. Using dry milk solids or cottage cheese in a recipe can help mimic glutenous structure. Sometimes using the moisture tricks listed above will also solve structure problems with products that come out too dense and crumbly. It's important to avoid over-kneading or -beating gluten-free dough, as there is no gluten to develop with kneading.

Substitutions

Butter

Try to use butter substitutes that come as a stick, rather than in a tub as these will contain a similar amount of moisture than regular butter. Shortening, coconut oil, olive oil and silken tofu are all suitable substitutes. Using combinations of these ingredients will work best.

Eggs

Store bought egg replacer is a good option for substitution. Alternative ingredients include milled flax seeds, silken tofu, mashed bananas or figs. Milk can also work if boosting with additional baking powder. If using flax seed, it must be milled and combined with hot water before using.

Milk

Coconut, soy, rice and nut milks can be substituted for regular milk.

Sugar

3/4 cup honey can be substituted for 1 cup of granulated or brown sugar, if liquid in the recipe is reduced by 1/4 cup. Maple syrup, brown rice syrup and agave can also be used instead of honey.

Roasted stone fruits with vanilla

Ingredients

- 175g golden caster sugar

- 1 vanilla pod, split in two

- 5 cardamom pods

- zest and juice 1 lime

- 6 apricots, halved and stoned

- 3 peaches, quartered and stoned

- 3 nectarines, quartered and stoned

Directions

• STEP 1

Heat oven to 220C/fan 200C/gas 8. Tip the sugar, vanilla pod, cardamom, lime zest and juice into a food processor, then blitz until blended, or mash together using a pestle and mortar. Tip the fruit into a shallow baking dish, then toss in the sludgy sugar.

• STEP 2

Roast for 20 mins until the fruits have softened, but not collapsed and the sugar and fruit juices have made a sticky sauce. Any leftovers will keep in the fridge for up to 2 days.

Banana, clementine & mango smoothie

Ingredients

• about 24 juicy clementines, plus an extra one for decoration

• 2 small, very ripe and juicy mangoes

• 2 ripe bananas

• 500g tub whole milk or low-fat yogurt

• handful of ice cubes (optional)

Directions

• STEP 1

Halve the clementines and squeeze out the juice –
you should have about 600ml/1 pint. (This can be
done the night before.) Peel the mangoes, slice the
fruit away from the stone in the centre, then chop
the flesh into rough pieces. Peel and slice the
bananas.

• STEP 2

Put the clementine juice, mango flesh, bananas,
yogurt and ice cubes into a liquidiser and blend
until smooth. Pour into six glasses and serve. (You
might need to make this in two batches, depending
on the size of your liquidiser.) If you don't add ice
cubes, chill in the fridge until ready to serve.

Hash browns with gruyère & pancetta

Ingredients

- 800g Maris Piper or King Edward potatoes

- 1 ½ tbsp olive oil

- 1 small onion, finely diced

- 2 garlic cloves

- 75g pancetta, diced

- 50g gruyère, grated

- small pack parsley, chopped

- 2 large eggs, lightly beaten

- roasted cherry tomatoes and mushrooms, to serve (optional)

Directions

- STEP 1

Peel the potatoes, cut them into large chunks and put them in a saucepan of cold salted water. Bring to the boil and simmer for 15 mins until just cooked (do not overcook or the potatoes will absorb too much water).

- STEP 2

Meanwhile, heat 1/2 tbsp of the olive oil in a small pan. Add the onion, garlic and a pinch of salt, then cover and cook over a low heat for 15-20 mins until the onion is soft and starting to caramelise. If the onion starts to catch, add a splash of cold water. Remove the onion and garlic, then fry the pancetta in the same pan until the fat has melted and the pancetta is crisp.

- STEP 3

Drain the potatoes and allow to steam-dry. Once cool enough to handle, chop the potatoes into 1cm dice and mix in a bowl with the pancetta, gruyère, parsley, beaten eggs, onion and garlic. Season generously with black pepper.

• STEP 4

Heat 1 tbsp of the oil in a large non-stick frying pan. Gently tip in the potato mixture and press down with the back of a large spoon. Fry over a medium heat for 15 mins until the bottom is golden brown. Tip the hash brown onto a plate, then slide back into the pan, cooked-side up. Cook for another 15 mins until golden and hot. Serve with roasted tomatoes and mushrooms, if you like.

Mango & passion fruit smoothie

Ingredients

- 400g/14oz peeled and chopped ripe mango

- 2 x 125g pots fat-free mango yogurt

- 250ml skimmed milk

- juice 1 lime

- 4 passion fruits, halved

Directions

- STEP 1

Whizz the mango, yogurt and milk together in a blender until smooth. Stir in the lime juice, then pour into 4 glasses. Scoop the pulp of a passion fruit into each one, and swirl before serving.

Oven-baked egg & chips

Ingredients

• 2 medium baking potatoes, cut into chunky wedges

• 2 tbsp olive oil

• 1 tsp smoked paprika

• 2 tomatoes, halved

• 2 eggs

Directions

• STEP 1

Heat oven to 190C/170C fan/gas 5. Tip the potato wedges into a roasting tin. Drizzle over the oil and sprinkle over the paprika. Season and mix well to coat the potatoes. Roast for 25 mins, turning halfway through, until almost tender.

• STEP 2

Nestle the tomatoes, cut-side up, amongst the potatoes. Make 2 spaces in the tin and crack an egg into each one. Return to the oven for 6-8 mins until the eggs are just set.

Sprout & spinach baked eggs

Ingredients

• 1 tbsp olive oil

- 1 tsp cumin seeds

- 1 onion, chopped

- 2 garlic cloves, crushed

- 1 green chilli, chopped (deseeded if you don't want it very hot)

- 300g brussels sprouts, roughly shredded

- 450g spinach

- ½ lemon, juiced

- 6 eggs

- ½ small pack coriander, yogurt, sriracha and thick slices of sourdough or keto bread, to serve

Directions

• STEP 1

Heat the oil in a frying pan with high sides, scatter in the cumin seeds and toast a little, then add the onion and fry until softened, around 5 mins. Add the garlic and chilli and fry for 1 min. Tip the sprouts into the pan and cook for 5 mins until softened, then add the spinach – you may have to do this in batches. Cook until the spinach has wilted down, then squeeze in the lemon juice to taste. Season well.

• STEP 2

Use a spoon to create six holes in the greens to crack the eggs into. Break the eggs into the holes, cover the pan with a lid and cook for 5-7 mins until the eggs have set, but the yolk remains runny.

Sprinkle over the coriander and serve immediately, drizzled with natural yogurt and sriracha, and with sourdough or keto bread on the side.

Fruit & seed yogurt

Ingredients

• 1 sliced kiwi fruit

• 1 tsp mixed seeds

• ¼ tsp cinnamon

• 150g pot of 0% fat probiotic yogurt

Directions

• STEP 1

Stir the sliced kiwi, mixed seeds and cinnamon into the yogurt, and serve.

Instant berry banana slush

Ingredients

• 2 ripe bananas

• 200g frozen berry mix (blackberries, raspberries and currants)

Directions

• STEP 1

Slice the bananas into a bowl and add the frozen berry mix. Blitz with a stick blender to make a slushy ice and serve straight away in two glasses with spoons.

Veggie breakfast bakes

Ingredients

• 4 large field mushrooms

• 8 tomatoes, halved

• 1 garlic clove, thinly sliced

• 2 tsp olive oil

• 200g bag spinach

• 4 eggs

Directions

• STEP 1

Heat oven to 200C/180C fan/gas 6. Put the mushrooms and tomatoes into 4 ovenproof dishes. Divide garlic between the dishes, drizzle over the oil and some seasoning, then bake for 10 mins.

• STEP 2

Meanwhile, put the spinach into a large colander, then pour over a kettle of boiling water to wilt it. Squeeze out any excess water, then add the spinach to the dishes. Make a little gap between the vegetables and crack an egg into each dish. Return to the oven and cook for a further 8-10 mins or until the egg is cooked to your liking.

Sweet potato pancakes with orange & grapefruit

Ingredients

- 325g sweet potatoes, peeled and coarsely grated

- ½ tsp vanilla extract

- 2 oranges, 1 zested, both cut into segments

- 150g ricotta or bio yogurt

- 2 large eggs

- ½ tsp baking powder

- 2 tsp rapeseed oil

- 2 grapefruits, cut into segments

- small handful mint leaves

Directions

- STEP 1

Put the sweet potato in a bowl, cover with cling film and cook in the microwave on high for 5 mins (or steam them). Mash the potato with a fork. When cooled a little, beat in the vanilla, orange zest, ricotta, eggs and baking powder to make a batter.

• STEP 2

Heat the oil in a non-stick frying pan and fry spoonfuls of the batter for a few mins. Carefully flip the pancakes to cook the other side. When done, set aside on a plate and cook the remaining batter, aiming for eight pancakes in total. Serve when done.

Cloud eggs

Ingredients

• 2 large eggs

• 2 tbsp chives, chopped

• 2 spring onions, finely sliced

• wholemeal toast or gluten-free alternative, to serve (optional)

Directions

• STEP 1

Heat oven to 230C/210C fan/gas 8. Separate the egg whites from the yolks. Tip the whites into a large, clean mixing bowl and beat with an electric whisk until aerated and fluffy.

• STEP 2

Gently fold through 1½ tbsp of the chives and the spring onion. Line a baking sheet with baking parchment, then pile on the egg whites in two mounds. Use the back of a spoon to make a dip in the centre of each one. Bake for 8-10 mins until set and turning light golden brown. Gently tip the egg yolk into the centre of the egg whites and return to the oven for a further 2-3 mins, or until the yolk has just set. Serve sprinkled with the remaining chives. Eat on toast, or just as they come.

Tropical breakfast smoothie

Ingredients

- 3 passion fruits

- 1 banana, chopped

- 1small mango, peeled, stoned and chopped

- 300ml orange juice

- ice cubes

Directions

- STEP 1

Scoop the pulp of the passion fruits into a blender and add the banana, mango and orange juice. Purée until smooth and drink immediately, topped with ice cubes.

Blueberry smoothie recipe

Ingredients

- 175g blueberries

- 1 small banana, sliced

- 1 tbsp natural or Greek yogurt

- 100ml apple juice, chilled

- 3-4 mint leaves (optional), plus extra to garnish

Directions

- STEP 1

Put the blueberries, banana, yogurt, apple juice and mint, if using, in a blender and blitz until smooth. Add a splash of water if it seems too thick.

- STEP 2

Pour the smoothie into a tall glass with a glass straw to serve. Garnish with a sprig of mint, if you like.

Crispy hash browns

Ingredients

• 3 medium-sized potatoes (approx. 370g in total, unpeeled, left whole – Maris Pipers, King Edward and Desirée are all good choices)

• 50g butter, melted

• 4 tbsp sunflower oil

Directions

• STEP 1

Cook the potatoes in a saucepan of boiling water for 10 mins then drain and set aside until cool enough to handle.

• STEP 2

Coarsely grate the potatoes into a bowl discarding any skin that comes off in your hand as you grate. Season well with salt and pepper and pour over half the butter. Mix well then divide the mix into 8 and shape into patties or squares. The hash browns can be prepared a day ahead and chilled until ready to cook or frozen for up to a month.

• STEP 3

To cook, heat the oil and the remaining butter in a frying pan until sizzling and gently fry the hash browns, in batches if needed, for 4-5 mins on each side until crisp and golden. Serve straight away or leave in a low oven to keep warm.

CHAPTER 5
LOW FODMAP, HIGH FIBER, GLUTEN FREE DIET RECIPES FOR LUNCH

Rustic beans & spinach with garlic yogurt

Ingredients

- 2 tbsp rapeseed oil

- 1 large onion, halved and sliced

- 170g carrots, cut into small chunks

- 5 garlic cloves, 3 finely sliced and 2 crushed

- 1 tbsp sherry vinegar

- 1 red pepper, deseeded and chopped

- ½ tsp vegetable bouillon powder, made up to 250ml with boiling water

- 2 rosemary sprigs

- 1 tbsp smoked paprika, plus a pinch to serve

- 150g whole cherry tomatoes

- 1 ½ tbsp tomato purée

- 400g and 210g cans butter beans, drained

- 2 x 120g pots bio yogurt

- 160g baby spinach

- squeeze lemon (optional)

Instructions

• STEP 1

Heat the oil in a large pan and fry the onion, carrots and sliced garlic, stirring frequently for 10 mins until the veg starts to caramelise. Pour in the sherry vinegar, allowing it to sizzle in the heat, then add the pepper, bouillon, rosemary, paprika, cherry tomatoes, tomato purée and beans, and cook for 15 mins. Meanwhile, stir the yogurt and crushed garlic together.

• STEP 2

Stir the spinach into the pan and cook until wilted, adding a splash of water if you need to. Add some lemon juice to taste if you like, then serve in bowls topped with a dollop of the yogurt, a pinch of paprika and a good grinding of black pepper.

Cumin-spiced chicken with squash

Ingredients

- 150ml bio-yogurt

- 1 tbsp finely grated ginger

- ½ tsp ground turmeric

- 1 tsp ground cumin

- 4 skinless chicken thighs fillets (about 250g), cut into big chunks

- 200g butternut squash, cut into bite-sized chunks (no need to peel)

- 1 tbsp coconut oil

- 2 red onions, halved and thickly sliced

- 1 garlic clove

- 4 sprigs mint, leaves picked

- 25g coriander, chopped

- 300g can red kidney beans, drained and rinsed

- grated zest and juice 0.5 lime

- 1 head of chicory, thickly sliced

Instructions

- STEP 1

Put 2 tbsp of the yogurt in a bowl with the spices, chicken and a really good grinding of black pepper, and set aside for 30 mins, or longer if you have time, to marinate.

• STEP 2

Heat oven to 200C/180C fan/gas 6. Arrange the squash on a large baking tray, crumble over the coconut oil (as it will be solid at this stage) and roast for 20 mins. Add the onions and chicken, spaced apart, and roast for 20 mins more until everything is cooked.

• STEP 3

Meanwhile, put the rest of the yogurt in a bowl with the garlic, mint and two-thirds of the coriander, and blitz with a hand blender until smooth. Tip the beans and remaining coriander into a bowl, and add the lime zest and juice with a couple of tbsp of the yogurt dressing. Tip in the squash, onions and chicken, add the chicory and toss everything together. Pile onto plates and drizzle with the remaining dressing. (If eating cold as a packed lunch, take the dressing in a pot and dress the salad when ready to eat.)

Spicy tuna quinoa salad

Ingredients

• 1 onion, sliced

• 350g pepper, sliced

• 1 tbsp olive oil

• 1 red chilli, finely chopped

• 225g pouch ready-to-eat quinoa

- 350g cherry tomato, halved

- handful black olives, chopped

- 225g jar albacore tuna in olive oil, flaked

Instructions

- STEP 1

Fry the onion and peppers in the oil until soft. Add the chilli and cool slightly.

- STEP 2

Mix the quinoa, onion mixture, cherry tomatoes, olives and tuna together. Divide between 4 plates, pour over a little of the oil from the tuna jar, season and serve.

Potato frittata with pepper salsa

Ingredients

• 1 kg even-sized potatoes, peeled and thinly sliced

• 8 eggs

• 2 red chillies

• 3 garlic cloves, finely grated

• 4 handfuls of rocket

For the salsa

• 1 tsp rapeseed oil, plus extra for the dish

• 2 red peppers, halved and deseeded

* 325g can sweetcorn, drained

* 1 red onion, finely chopped

* handful of basil (about 10g), roughly chopped

* ½ tsp lime zest and 1 tbsp juice

Instructions

• STEP 1

Heat the oven to 220C/200C fan/gas 7. Boil the potatoes for 5 mins until just cooked, then drain. Meanwhile, beat the eggs in a bowl with the chillies, garlic and lots of black pepper. For the salsa, lightly oil the pepper halves and place, cut-side down, on a baking sheet.

• STEP 2

Stir the potatoes into the egg mixture, then tip into a shallow, lightly oiled ovenproof dish (ours was a deep 30cm dish). Cook in the oven with the peppers on the shelf above for 25-30 mins until the egg is set and starting to brown at the edges.

• STEP 3

Meanwhile, tip the sweetcorn into a bowl with the onion and basil, and stir in the lime zest and juice. Peel the roasted peppers, dice the flesh, and add to make the salsa.

• STEP 4

Serve half the frittata with half the salsa and half the rocket for two people. The remainder will keep chilled for up to three days. Serve cold or lightly warmed with the remaining salsa.

Air-fryer boiled eggs

Ingredients

* 6 eggs

* toast, to serve (optional)

Instructions

* STEP 1

Heat the air-fryer to 180C. Put the eggs in the air-fryer basket and cook, in one layer, for 8-14 mins – nearer to 8 mins will be soft-boiled, while 14 mins will be hard-boiled.

* STEP 2

Put the eggs in a bowl of ice cold water briefly to stop them from cooking. Peel or serve in egg cups with toast on the side, if you like.

Vegan nuggets

Ingredients

- 300g cauliflower florets (or ¾ small cauliflower)

- 2 carrots, chopped (about 165g)

- ½ medium onion, chopped

- 1 tbsp olive oil

- 1 garlic clove, crushed

- 2 tbsp nutritional yeast

- 2 tsp yeast extract

- 400g can cannellini beans, drained

- 50g gram (chickpea) flour

- olive oil, for the baking tray

For the coating

- 100g gram flour, plus a little extra

- 100g breadcrumbs (gluten-free if necessary)

- ½ tsp mustard powder

- ½ tsp onion powder

- ½ tsp garlic powder

Instructions

• STEP 1

Pulse the cauliflower, carrots and onion in a food processor until very finely chopped, like rice. Heat the oil in a large frying pan and gently fry the mix for 12-15 mins until softened. Add the garlic and fry for a further 1 min, then take off the heat and stir in the nutritional yeast and yeast extract. Set aside.

• STEP 2

Blend the beans into a mushy purée in a food processor, then add to the veggie mix and combine well. Stir in the flour and season. Put in the fridge to firm up for 1 hr.

• STEP 3

Heat the oven to 220C/200C fan/gas 7. Line a large baking tray with baking parchment and coat with a little olive oil. To make the coating, mix the gram flour with 150ml water using a fork so it resembles beaten egg, then season. Scatter the extra gram flour on a plate. Mix the breadcrumbs with the spices and scatter onto a second plate.

• STEP 4

Roll the bean mixture into walnut-sized pieces, then flatten to form nugget shapes. Dip the pieces first in the gram flour, then in the gram batter, and finally roll in the breadcrumbs – handle carefully as they will be a little soft. When the nuggets are fully coated, lay them out on the prepared tray.

• STEP 5

Bake for 20 mins, then use tongs to turn each nugget over and bake for a further 15 mins until they are dark golden and crisp. Leave to cool for 20 mins before serving with your choice of dipping sauces.

Prawn & avocado wrap

Ingredients

• 1 very ripe baby avocado, stoned, peeled and roughly chopped

• juice ½ lime

• few shakes Tabasco sauce

• 1 tomato, deseeded and chopped

• 1 spring onion, sliced

- 1 seeded flour tortilla (or gluten-free alternative)

- handful mixed salad leaves

- 85g cooked and peeled prawn

Instructions

- STEP 1

Put the avocado in a bowl with the lime juice, Tabasco and some seasoning. Roughly mash, then add the tomato, coriander (if using) and spring onion.

- STEP 2

Warm the wrap in the microwave for a few seconds. Spread the avocado mixture down the middle, scatter on the salad leaves and finish with the prawns. Roll up, then eat.

Lebanese-style meatballs with mujadara

Ingredients

• 250g lamb mince (10% fat or lower)

• 2 large onions (320g), 1 very finely chopped, 1 halved and thinly sliced

• 1 garlic clove, finely grated

• 3 tsp ground cumin

• 1 lemon, half zested and juiced, half cut into four wedges to serve

• 2 tsp rapeseed oil

- 200g brown basmati rice

- 1 tbsp bouillon powder

- 390g can green lentils, drained

- 2 tbsp tahini

For the salad

- 4 tomatoes, cut into wedges

- ¼ cucumber (about 150g), sliced

- 12 Kalamata olives, quartered

- 1 tbsp chopped mint, plus a few small leaves to serve

Instructions

• STEP 1

Tip the lamb into a bowl with ¼ of the chopped onion, the garlic, ½ tsp cumin, the lemon zest and some black pepper. Mix well with your hands, then shape into 16 small meatballs. Chill for at least 30 mins.

• STEP 2

Heat 1 tsp oil in a non-stick frying pan over a medium-high heat. Reserve most of the remaining chopped onion for the salad, then fry the rest for 5 mins until golden. Stir in the remaining cumin, then tip in the rice, bouillon powder, 500ml water and some black pepper. Reduce the heat to a simmer, then cover and cook over a medium heat for 30 mins. Tip in the lentils, cover again and cook for 5-10 mins more until the rice is tender and all the water has been absorbed.

• STEP 3

Meanwhile, heat the remaining oil in a non-stick pan over a medium-high heat. Add the meatballs and sliced onion, cover and cook for 5 mins. Stir, then cook for 5 mins more until the meatballs are cooked through and the onions are golden. Stir the tahini and lemon juice together with 3-4 tbsp water to make a sauce.

• STEP 4

Mix all of the salad Ingredients with the reserved chopped onion. Serve.

Tomato, watermelon & feta salad with mint dressing

Ingredients

- 2 tbsp olive oil

- 1 tbsp red wine vinegar

- ¼ tsp chilli flakes

- 2 tbsp chopped mint

- 4 tomatoes, chopped

- 500g/1lb 2oz watermelon, cut into chunks

- 200g pack feta cheese, crumbled

Instructions

- STEP 1

Make the dressing by mixing the oil, vinegar, chilli flakes and mint with some seasoning.

- STEP 2

Put the tomatoes and watermelon in a bowl. Pour over the dressing and leave to stand for 10 mins to allow the fruit to get really juicy. Gently stir through the feta, then serve.

Roasted summer vegetable casserole

Ingredients

- 3 tbsp olive oil

- 1 garlic bulb, halved through the middle

* 2 large courgettes, thickly sliced

* 1 large red onion, sliced

* 1 aubergine, halved and sliced on the diagonal

* 2 large tomatoes, quartered

* 200g new potatoes, scrubbed and halved

* 1 red pepper, deseeded and cut into chunky pieces

* 400g can chopped tomatoes

* 0.5 small pack parsley, chopped

Instructions

* STEP 1

Heat oven to 200C/180C fan/gas 6 and put the oil in a roasting tin. Tip in the garlic and all the fresh veg, then toss with your hands to coat in the oil. Season well and roast for 45 mins.

• STEP 2

Remove the garlic from the roasting tin and squeeze out the softened cloves all over the veg, stirring to evenly distribute. In a medium pan, simmer the chopped tomatoes until bubbling, season well and stir through the roasted veg in the tin. Scatter over the parsley and serve.

Bean & quinoa salad with orange

Ingredients

• 120g quinoa

- 320g celery, strings removed if tough, sliced

- 320g frozen soya beans

- 2 tbsp extra virgin olive oil

- 3 tbsp apple cider vinegar

- 8 spring onions, trimmed and thinly sliced

- 30g flat-leaf parsley, chopped

- 4 tbsp chopped mint (optional)

- 4 small oranges, peeled and segmented

- 120g feta, crumbled

Instructions

- STEP 1

Tip the quinoa and celery into a pan and cover with plenty of water. Bring to the boil, then reduce the heat and simmer for 10 mins. Add the soya beans, bring back to the boil and cook for 7 mins more. Drain well, tip into a bowl and set aside.

• STEP 2

Add the oil, vinegar and spring onions, and leave to cool slightly before stirring in the parsley and mint. Serve two portions topped with half the segmented oranges and half the feta crumbled over. Chill the remaining salad for another day, then segment the remaining oranges and crumble over the feta just before serving. Will keep chilled in an airtight container for up to three days.

Tuna, avocado & pea salad in Baby Gem lettuce wraps

Ingredients

• 1 ½ tbsp low-fat natural yogurt

• 85g canned tuna chunks (in spring water), drained

• 50g cooked and cooled rice (use leftover from Prawn, butternut & mango curry dinner if made - see 'goes well with', right)

• 85g frozen pea, cooked, then refreshed in cold water

• ½ red pepper, chopped

• 1 avocado, stoned, peeled and cut into chunks

• zest and juice 1 lime

• small pack coriander, chopped

• 1 large Baby Gem lettuce, or other crisp lettuce, such as cos

Instructions

• STEP 1

Combine all the Ingredients except the lettuce in a bowl, season, then chill until ready to eat. Spoon the tuna mix on top of the lettuce leaves, wrap up and enjoy.

Watermelon, prawn & avocado salad

Ingredients

* 1 small red onion, finely chopped

* 1 fat garlic clove, crushed

* 1 small red chilli, finely chopped

* juice 1 lime

* 1 tbsp rice or white wine vinegar

* 1 tsp caster sugar

* watermelon wedge, deseeded and diced

* 1 avocado, diced

* small bunch coriander leaves, chopped

* 200g cooked tiger prawns, defrosted if frozen

Instructions

- STEP 1

Put the onion in a medium bowl with the garlic, chilli, lime juice, vinegar, sugar and some seasoning. Leave to marinate for 10 mins.

- STEP 2

Add the watermelon, avocado, coriander and prawns, then toss gently to serve.

Smoked mackerel & beetroot salad with creamy horseradish dressing

Ingredients

- 6-10 beetroots (depending on size)

- 140g puy lentils, cooked

• bunch spring onions (about 8), sliced on an angle

• 1 eating apple, core removed, thinly sliced (squeeze a little lemon juice over to prevent them turning brown)

• 1 small radicchio, leaves separated and torn into bite-sized chunks

• 1 pack smoked mackerel (approx 250g), skin and any bones removed, flaked into chunky pieces

For the horseradish dressing

• zest and juice 1 lemon

• 150ml pot soured cream

• 2 tbsp creamed horseradish

Instructions

• STEP 1

Heat oven to 200C/180C fan/gas 6. Place the unpeeled beetroots on a baking tray and roast for 35-50 mins, depending on their size. Give them a gentle squeeze after 35 mins – if they feel tender and are a little shrivelled, they are done; if not, continue cooking. Remove from the oven and set aside to cool.

• STEP 2

Using a small sharp knife, carefully peel the beetroots, then cut into wedges (wear plastic gloves to prevent them staining your hands). Mix the dressing Ingredients in a small bowl. Put the lentils, spring onions, apple, radicchio and mackerel in a large bowl, add half the dressing and toss everything together. Pile the Ingredients onto a serving platter, layering with the beetroots as you do. Serve with the remaining dressing on the side.

Alu tamatar masala

Ingredients

- 6 medium potatoes (about 1kg), roughly chopped

- 2 tbsp sunflower oil

- 1 tsp black mustard seeds

- 6-8 curry leaves

- 1 green chilli, thinly sliced

- 2 garlic cloves, finely chopped

- 2.5cm piece of ginger, peeled and finely chopped

- 5 medium tomatoes, finely chopped

- 1 tsp garam masala

- ½ tsp chilli powder

- ½ tsp ground turmeric

- handful of coriander leaves

Instructions

- STEP 1

Bring a large pan of water to the boil over a medium-high heat and cook the potatoes for 10-15 mins until just tender (a cutlery knife should just be able to cut through). Drain and set aside.

- STEP 2

Heat the oil in a large frying pan over a low heat and add the mustard seeds. When they begin to pop, add the curry leaves, chilli, garlic and ginger, and cook for 1 min until the aromas start to release. Stir in the tomatoes, then cover and cook for 10 mins until soft and mushy

- STEP 3

Add the garam masala, chilli powder, turmeric and 1 tsp salt. Mix well and cook for another minute before adding the cooked potatoes. Pour in 200ml water, cover and simmer for 10 mins until the potatoes are completely tender. Mash a few of the potatoes with a potato masher, keeping the rest whole. Sprinkle over the coriander leaves to serve.

Air-fryer turkey crown

Ingredients

- 1.7kg turkey crown

- 1 tsp vegetable oil

- 1 tsp dried mixed herbs

- 1 clementine, halved

- 1 shallot, halved

- 2 garlic cloves, bashed

- a few fresh herb sprigs, such as sage, thyme or oregano

Instructions

• STEP 1

Heat the air fryer using its preheat function, or set to 180C for 2 mins. Pat the turkey crown dry using kitchen paper, then rub all over with the oil. Season well, then scatter the dried herbs over the skin. If the crown allows, stuff the clementine halves, shallot, garlic cloves and fresh herb sprigs into the cavity. If this is not possible, tuck them around the crown in the air-fryer basket instead. Either way, ensure the turkey crown is skin-side down in the air-fryer basket.

• STEP 2

Cook for 30 mins, then turn the crown over and cook for a further 20-30 mins, or until the juices run clear when pierced with a knife in the thickest part, or a meat thermometer stuck reads 65C. Carve into slices to serve.

Chorizo & chickpea summer stew

Ingredients

• 1 tbsp olive oil

• 2 garlic cloves, crushed

• 2 thyme sprigs

• 1 tbsp smoked paprika

• 200g chorizo ring, sliced into thin coins

• 1 tbsp sherry vinegar

• 600g cherry tomatoes, halved

• 450g jar roasted red peppers, drained and cut into large strips

• 100g spinach

• 2 x 400g cans chickpeas, drained

• drizzle of extra virgin olive oil and crusty bread, to serve

Instructions

• STEP 1

Heat the oil in a large frying pan over a medium heat, add the garlic, thyme and smoked paprika, and stir for a few minutes, then tip in the chorizo and stir for another couple of minutes until its oil is released. Splash in the sherry vinegar and let it bubble for a minute or so.

- STEP 2

Add the tomatoes, peppers, spinach and chickpeas along with 100ml water and a pinch of seasoning. Bring to the boil, then reduce the heat to a simmer and cook until the tomatoes have softened and there is a thickened sauce, about 15 mins. Adjust the seasoning and finish with a drizzle of extra virgin olive oil. Serve with crusty bread.

Poached chicken breast

Ingredients

- 1 carrot, roughly sliced

- 1 celery stick, roughly chopped

- 3 large garlic cloves

- ½ small bunch parsley

- ½ small bunch dill

- 4 skinless chicken breasts

- 1l cold water

Instructions

- STEP 1

Tip the carrot, celery and garlic into a large saucepan. Tie the herbs together in a bunch with a piece of kitchen string, then add to the pan with the chicken breasts, water and 2 tsp salt (adding a little more water if it doesn't quite cover the chicken). Bring to the boil, then immediately lower to a simmer and cook over a very low heat for 15 mins, or until the juices run clear in the thickest part of the breast.

• STEP 2

Remove the pan from the heat and scoop out the chicken breasts from the poaching liquid. Wrap the chicken in tin foil and leave to rest for 5 mins. Slice or tear the chicken into pieces and use in salads, soups or sandwiches.

Toddler recipe: Microwave courgette and pea risotto with prawns

Ingredients

• 200g risotto rice

• 1 large garlic clove, crushed

* 2 spring onions, finely sliced

* 900ml low-salt chicken stock (we used gluten-free Kallo, see tips below)

* 120g frozen peas

* 1 large courgette, diced (see tips below)

* 50g grated medium or mature cheddar, plus extra to serve

* 140g cooked prawns (or chicken)

Instructions

* STEP 1

Put the rice, garlic and spring onions into a large microwaveable bowl, then pour in 400ml stock.

Cover with cling film and microwave on High for 10 mins. Stir the rice, then add another 250ml of the remaining stock, cover and microwave on High again for 3 mins.

• STEP 2

Stir the rice again, then add the frozen peas, courgette and the rest of the stock. Cover and microwave on the same setting for a further 8 mins. Stir in the cheese and prawns (or chicken if you prefer), then leave the risotto to stand for 2 mins. Scatter with more cheese and serve.

Fennel, cherry & goat's cheese salad with lentils

Ingredients

• 50g walnut halves or pieces

- 250g pack pre-cooked puy lentils

- 1 large fennel bulb, finely sliced, fronds reserved

- 140g cherries, halved and pitted (or small figs, halved)

- 1 tbsp red wine vinegar

- 2 tbsp extra virgin olive oil

- 1 tsp Dijon mustard

- ½ tsp clear honey

- ½ small pack tarragon, roughly chopped

- 100g pack soft goat's cheese (any kind will work, but ash-rolled looks a bit special), thickly sliced and halved

Instructions

- STEP 1

Heat a dry frying pan over a low-medium heat. Add the walnuts and cook for 3 mins, stirring frequently, until they smell toasty and the skins are a deep golden brown. Set aside to cool.

- STEP 2

Heat the lentils following pack instructions, then tip into a large bowl and loosen with a fork. Tip the fennel and cherries on top.

- STEP 3

Whisk together the vinegar, oil, mustard, honey and tarragon, then season. Fold the dressing through the lentils, fennel and cherries, then scoop the salad onto a platter. Scatter with the cheese, walnuts and the reserved fennel fronds.

Vegan Thai green curry

Ingredients

• 200g baby potatoes, halved

• 100g green beans, trimmed and halved

• 1 tbsp rapeseed oil

• 1 garlic clove, finely sliced

• 1 tbsp Thai green curry paste (check the label to make sure it's vegetarian/ vegan)

• 400g can light coconut milk

* 1 lime, zest pared in thick strips

* 80g sugar snap peas, halved lengthways

* 150g cherry tomatoes, halved

* 100g firm tofu, chopped into small cubes

* small bunch coriander, chopped

* 200g jasmine rice, cooked following pack instructions

Instructions

* STEP 1

Cook the potatoes in boiling water for 8 mins. Add the green beans and cook for a further 3 mins, then drain.

• STEP 2

Heat the oil in a wok or pan, fry the garlic for 1 min, add the curry paste and cook for 1 min, or until it starts to darken a little and smell fragrant. Stir in the coconut milk and bring to a simmer, drop in the lime zest and gently bubble for 5 mins to thicken the sauce a little.

• STEP 3

Add the potatoes and beans followed by the sugar snap peas and cook for 1 min before stirring in the cherry tomatoes and tofu.

• STEP 4

Cut the lime in half and squeeze the juice into the pan, then stir in the coriander and serve over the rice.

Loaded potato skins with speedy baked beans

Ingredients

• 2 baking potatoes (about 250g each)

• drizzle of rapeseed oil

• 50g mature cheddar, finely grated

• 2 spring onions, white parts finely chopped (save the greens for another recipe)

For the beans

• ½ tsp rapeseed oil

• 2 garlic cloves, finely grated

• 2 tbsp tomato purée

• 1 tbsp balsamic vinegar

• 1 tsp smoked paprika

• 400g can cannellini beans

Instructions

• STEP 1

Heat the oven to 220C/200C fan/gas 7. Rub the potatoes with a small drop of the oil, then put on a baking tray and bake for 50 mins until almost tender. Toss the cheese and onion together and set aside.

• STEP 2

Meanwhile, make the beans. Heat the rest of the oil in a small non-stick pan and fry the garlic over a low heat for about a minute, stirring to soften. Add the tomato purée, vinegar and paprika, and cook, stirring, for about a minute more. Tip in the beans and the liquid from the can. Cook for a few minutes so the beans are coated in the sauce, then turn off the heat. Set aside until the potatoes are ready.

Air-fryer fish & chips

Ingredients

• 60g cornflour

• 1 tsp smoked paprika

• ½ tsp dried mixed herbs

• 2 white fish fillets, such as cod, haddock or basa

• 3 medium potatoes, such as Desirée or Maris Piper

• 6-8 tbsp vegetable oil

• mushy peas and tartar sauce, to serve (optional)

Instructions

• STEP 1

Mix together the cornflour, paprika and mixed herbs with 1 tsp salt and ¼ tsp freshly ground black pepper and spread out on a large dinner plate. Coat the fish fillets in the flour mixture on both sides. If you prefer to cook on the hob, see tip below – the fish fillets are now ready to fry.

• STEP 2

Cut the potatoes into 1cm-thick chips using a large, sharp knife. Leave the skin on, or peel them, if you like.

• STEP 3

Put the chips in a large mixing bowl, then add 2 tbsp of the vegetable oil and a good pinch of salt and pepper. Toss until well coated. Set the air-fryer to 200C and cook the chips for around 18-22 mins, turning halfway (or shake the air-fryer basket) until crisp and cooked. Alternatively, you can cook them in the oven (see tip, below). Keep warm while you cook the fish or cook it in the second air-fryer basket, if you have one.

• STEP 4

Spread 4 tbsp of the vegetable oil out on a large dinner plate and dredge the coated fish in the oil to cover. Set the air-fryer to 200C and cook for 8-10 mins (depending on the size of your fish fillets), carefully turning halfway. Serve with mushy peas and tartar sauce, if you like. If freezing the fish and chips, defrost fully in the fridge, then reheat in the oven until piping hot.

Recipe tips

To cook the fish on the hob: Place a frying pan over a medium heat with enough oil to coat the bottom of the pan in a thin layer. Once the oil is hot, carefully place the coated fillets in the pan – they should sizzle slightly. Fry on each side until crisp and golden – about 3-4 mins on each side. Transfer to a plate lined with kitchen paper to drain the excess oil.

To cook the chips in the oven: Heat the oven to 220C/200C fan/gas 7. Put the chips in a pan of boiling water for 3 mins. Drain, then oil a large baking tray (use about 4 tbsp). Tip the chips into the tray, season with salt and pepper, and turn until well coated. Cook for 20-25 mins, turning halfway, until golden.

Honeyed harissa cod with crispy chickpeas

Ingredients

• 400g can chickpeas, rinsed and drained

• 1 tbsp olive oil

• 4 tbsp runny honey

• 2 tbsp harissa

* 1 garlic clove, crushed

* ½ thumb-sized piece ginger, finely grated

* 2 cod fillets or other sustainable firm white fish

* 120g green beans or long-stem broccoli, trimmed

Instructions

* STEP 1

Heat the oven to 220C/200C fan/gas 7. Pat the chickpeas dry with kitchen paper, and tip into a small roasting tin with the oil. Season well and toss together. Cook for 15 minutes, tossing occasionally, until the chickpeas start to crisp up and split.

* STEP 2

Mix the runny honey, harissa, garlic and ginger in a small bowl. Season the fish with salt and pepper, and add to the chickpeas in the roasting tin. Spoon over most of the dressing and bake for another 6-8 mins until the fish is flaky when pressed, and cooked through.

• STEP 3

While the fish is baking, cook the beans in boiling salted water for 4-6 mins until just tender. Serve over the chickpeas alongside the fish, with the remaining harissa-honey dressing on the side to serve.

Beef & swede casserole

Ingredients

- 2 tbsp vegetable oil

- 2 onions, sliced

- ½ celery stick, sliced

- 500g diced braising beef

- 200ml red wine (optional)

- 700ml beef stock (or chicken)

- 500g swede, peeled and cut into chunky dice

- 300g floury potatoes (such as Maris Piper), diced

- 3 thyme sprigs

- 1 bay leaf

- green vegetables, to serve (optional)

Instructions

- STEP 1

Heat the oil in a flameproof casserole dish over a medium-high heat. Fry the onions and celery for a few mins until turning brown. Add the beef and brown all over for 3-4 mins. Pour in the wine, if using, and let it reduce by half. Add the stock and toss in the swede, potatoes, thyme and bay leaf. Season and bring to the boil.

- STEP 2

Reduce the heat, cover with a lid and leave for 1 hr. If you want to reduce the liquid a little, remove the lid, turn up the heat and cook for a further 10-15 mins or until the sauce has thickened.

- STEP 3

Season to taste and remove the thyme sprigs and bay leaf. Serve with some green veg, if you like.

Turkey, courgetti & feta burgers

Ingredients

• 500g lean turkey mince

• 100g feta, crumbled

• 1 large courgette (about 200g), ends trimmed, halved widthways and spiralized into thin noodles

• 2 garlic cloves, crushed

• ½ small pack mint, leaves picked and chopped

• ½ tsp chilli flakes

* 1 tsp sumac

* zest and juice of 1 lemon (save the juice for the salad)

* 1 large egg, beaten

* 1 tsp olive oil

For the tomato salad

* 2 tbsp extra virgin olive oil

* 110g bag of rocket salad

* 250g pack cherry tomatoes, halved

Instructions

* STEP 1

Mix all of the Ingredients for the turkey burgers, bar the olive oil, together in a large bowl. Season with a generous amount of black pepper and a little salt (you won't need a lot because of the feta). Shape into 4 burgers, the mixture will be quite sticky so cover and chill in the fridge for 15 mins or until needed to firm up a little. At this point the burgers can also be frozen.

• STEP 2

Preheat the grill to its highest setting then brush the burgers on both sides with the olive oil. Transfer the burgers to a non-stick baking tray and cook for 8-10 mins on each side, until cooked through and golden brown.

• STEP 3

While the burgers are cooking, mix together the olive oil, lemon juice and some seasoning. Add the rocket and tomatoes to a large salad bowl, add half the dressing and toss well to combine. Serve alongside the turkey burgers and with the extra dressing on the side.

Cumin-spiced halloumi with corn & tomato slaw

Ingredients

- 1 lime, zested and juiced

- 1 tsp rapeseed oil

- 1 tsp fresh thyme leaves

- ¼ tsp turmeric

- ¼ tsp cumin seeds

- 1 tbsp finely chopped coriander

- 1 garlic clove, finely grated

- 100g halloumi, thinly sliced

For the slaw

- 1 lime, zested and juiced

- 3 tbsp bio yogurt

- 3 tbsp finely chopped coriander

- 1 red chilli, deseeded and chopped

- 160g corn, cut from 2 fresh cobs

- 1 red pepper, deseeded and chopped

• 100g fine green beans, blanched, trimmed and halved

• 200g cherry tomatoes, halved

• 1 red onion, halved and finely sliced

• 320g white cabbage, finely sliced

Instructions

• STEP 1

Mix the lime zest and juice with the oil, thyme, turmeric, cumin, coriander and garlic together in a bowl. Add the halloumi and carefully turn it until coated – take care as it breaks easily.

• STEP 2

To make the slaw, mix the lime juice and zest, yogurt, coriander and chilli together, then stir in the corn, red pepper, beans, tomatoes, onion and cabbage.

• STEP 3

Heat a large non-stick frying pan or griddle pan and fry the cheese in batches for 1 min each side. Serve the slaw on plates with the halloumi slices on top. If you're cooking for two people, serve half of the halloumi and slaw and chill the rest for lunch another day.

Korean clam broth - Jogaetang

Ingredients

• 500g medium-sized clams, rinsed (see below)

• 1 tbsp gochujang chilli paste or white miso if you don't want it to be spicy

• 2 large garlic cloves, finely chopped

• 3 spring onions, whites finely sliced, greens roughly chopped

• 2 handfuls beansprouts

• 1 green chilli, cut into matchsticks

• toasted sesame oil, to serve

• cooked rice, to serve

• kimchi or pickled cucumber, to serve

Instructions

• STEP 1

Drain the rinsed clams well and place them in a saucepan (with a lid) that fits them in a single layer. Pour over cold water to just cover (about 750ml should do it), then stir in the chilli paste, the garlic and the spring onion whites.

• STEP 2

Cover with a lid, bring to the boil, then turn down the heat and simmer gently for 2-3 mins until the clams have all opened. Turn off the heat and stir through the beansprouts and chilli. Season with salt to taste, and decant into one large or two smaller bowls. Top with the spring onion greens and a drizzle of sesame oil, and enjoy with rice and something sharp like kimchi or pickled cucumber.

You'll need soup spoons and a bowl for the empty
shells.

Vibrant spinach, coconut & paneer curry

Ingredients

• 2 tbsp oil or ghee

• 2 medium onions, sliced

• 4 garlic cloves, thinly sliced

• 1 tbsp ginger purée (roughly a thumb-sized
piece)

• small bunch of coriander, stalks finely chopped,
leaves picked

• 1½ tsp cumin seeds

- 1 tsp turmeric

- 1 green chilli, thinly sliced

- 400g coconut milk

- 200g spinach

- 250g paneer, cut into 2cm cubes

- ½ tsp garam masala

- ½ lemon, juiced

- cooked rice, to serve

Instructions

- STEP 1

Heat 1 tbsp of the oil or ghee in a large pan over a low-medium heat. Add the onions and sizzle for 15-20 mins until golden brown.

• STEP 2

Stir in the garlic, ginger, coriander stalks and cumin seeds. Turn up the heat a little and cook for a few minutes, stirring constantly, until the cumin seeds are aromatic, then add the turmeric, ½ the chilli, coconut milk (reserving 2 tbsp to serve) and spinach. If using fresh spinach, you may have to do this in batches, letting each handful wilt before adding the next. Season well, cover with a lid and cook for 5 mins, then remove the lid and bubble for another 5 mins.

• STEP 3

Meanwhile, heat the remaining oil or ghee in a frying pan and cook the paneer for 2-3 mins on each side until browned.

• STEP 4

Add half of the coriander leaves to the curry along with the garam masala and a squeeze of lemon juice, then take the pan off the heat and use a hand blender to blitz the curry until smooth and vibrant green. Add a splash of water if the sauce is too thick.

• STEP 5

Tip the paneer into the curry sauce and bubble for another minute. Serve scattered with the remaining chopped chilli and coriander leaves, then drizzle with the remaining coconut milk and serve with cooked rice.

CHAPTER 7
LOW FODMAP, HIGH FIBER, GLUTEN FREE DIET RECIPES FOR SNACKS

Sticky roasted parsnips, Chantenay carrots & apples

Ingredients

- 12 small parsnips, peeled and halved lengthways

- 600g Cantenay carrots

- 3 tbsp olive oil

- 2 tbsp clear honey

- 2 tsp coriander seeds, crushed

- 4 red eating apples, cored and quartered

Directions

• STEP 1

Heat oven to 180C/160C fan/gas 4. Put the parsnips and carrots in a large roasting tin. Mix the oil, honey and coriander seeds together with some seasoning and spoon over the vegetables, turning them to coat, then roast for 20 mins.

• STEP 2

Add the apples to the tin and cook for a further 20 mins until the vegetables are golden and just tender.

Mexican corn on the cob

Ingredients

* 4 corn cobs

* 100g butter, softened

* zest 1 lime

* 2 tsp chopped fresh chilli or 1 tsp chilli powder, mild or hot, depending how spicy you like it

* lime wedges, to serve

Directions

* STEP 1

Soak corn in cold water for 15 mins. Heat a griddle pan or barbecue and, when hot, place the corn directly on the bars. Cook for 30-40 mins, turning regularly, until the corn is tender and charred in spots.

• STEP 2

Meanwhile, mash the butter with the lime zest and chili. When the cobs are done, top each with a knob of flavoured butter and serve with lime wedges.

Pickled green beans

Ingredients

• 1kg green beans

• 140g coarse crystal sea salt

For the pickling vinegar

• 1 tbsp black peppercorns

• 1 tbsp coriander seeds

- 1 tbsp yellow mustard seeds

- 10 cloves

- few pieces of mace blades

- pinch of dried chilli flakes (optional)

- 2 bay leaves

- 700ml white wine vinegar, plus 3.5 tbsp

- 100g white sugar

- 1 finely chopped red onion

Directions

- STEP 1

Trim the stems from the green beans. In a large bowl, mix the coarse crystal sea salt with 300ml boiling water and let it dissolve to make a brining solution. Add 1.2 litres cold water, then the beans. Cover and leave to soak overnight, then rinse and drain.

• STEP 2

To make the pickling vinegar, put the whole spices in a medium saucepan. Toast over a low heat until they begin to smell aromatic. Add the dried chilli flakes last, as these can easily catch. Add the bay, pour in all of the vinegar, the sugar and the red onion, let the sugar dissolve, and bring to a simmer.

• STEP 3

Pack the beans into sterilised jars (see tip below), then pour over the hot vinegar and seal. Ready to eat in 2 weeks, or longer, if you like.

Perfect sushi rice

Ingredients

For the sushi-su

- 120ml rice vinegar or brown rice vinegar

- 3 tbsp sugar seasoning, to taste (optional)

- 1 tbsp sea salt

For the rice

- 450g Japanese rice (3 Japanese cups)

* 550g/ml water

Directions

* STEP 1

To make the rice, first wash it thoroughly in a sieve for 2 mins, gently turning it over by hand until the water runs clear. Drain the rice and put it in a pan with 550ml water.

* STEP 2

Leave it to stand for a minimum of 30 mins. It can be left overnight, but for best results, leave it for 30 mins-1 hr. Bring the water in the pan to the boil, put the lid on, reduce the heat and simmer for 8-9 mins. Turn the heat off and let it stand with the lid on for a further 5 mins. Do not lift the lid.

• STEP 3

While the rice is cooking, to make the sushi-su, put the rice vinegar, sugar and salt into a small container and mix with a spoon until the sugar and salt have dissolved.

• STEP 4

Put the rice into a wide flat dish such as a sushi oke, a baking dish or a roasting tray. Pour the sushi-su over the rice and fold it carefully in with a wooden spoon as it cools down, being careful not to damage the grains. You can use a fan or a hairdryer on the coolest setting to speed up the cooling process, directing it at the rice. The sushi-su gives the rice more flavour and that familiar sticky glazed look.

• STEP 5

If you don't want to use the rice immediately, cover it with a damp cloth so that it doesn't dry out. Leave in a cool place for up to 2 hrs. Do not refrigerate as the fridge will make the rice dry and hard to shape. Once assembled, the sushi can be chilled for a day.

Black beans & rice

Ingredients

• 250g basmati rice

• 2 x 400g cans black bean, drained and rinsed

Directions

• STEP 1

Put the rice in a large saucepan with a fitted lid. Cover with plenty of water and boil until al dente, about 8 mins. Drain and put back in the pan. Add the beans and stir through. Put the lid on and warm through for 5 mins before serving.

Brown-butter basted radishes & asparagus

Ingredients

• 100g unsalted butter

• 450g mixed radishes, larger ones sliced in half

• 450g pack asparagus, each spear chopped into 4 pieces

• juice ½ lemon, plus extra if needed

• 2 tbsp roughly chopped parsley

Directions

• STEP 1

Heat the butter gently in a non-stick frying pan. It will foam, then the solids will separate and begin to brown. This will take 15-20 mins – keep stirring, so that it doesn't blacken or burn.

• STEP 2

While the butter is browning, boil a large pan of salted water. Poach the radishes for 6 mins, then remove with a slotted spoon. Poach the asparagus for 2 mins, remove and put in iced water.

• STEP 3

Add the lemon juice to the butter, stir and keep over a very low heat while you add the radishes and drained asparagus. Baste them in the butter for 2 mins.

• STEP 4

Remove the vegetables from the browned butter and top with the parsley, plus a squeeze more lemon if you feel it needs it.

Crunchy parsnips

Ingredients

• 2kg parsnips, peeled, trimmed and cut into halves or quarters lengthways

• 100ml rapeseed or sunflower oil

• 5 tbsp polenta

• 2 tsp paprika

Directions

• STEP 1

Heat the oven to 220C/200C fan/gas 7. Blanch the parsnips in boiling water for 4-5 mins until slightly soft. Drain, leave to steam-dry, then tip into a large bowl. Drizzle over the oil and toss to coat all the parsnips.

• STEP 2

Mix the polenta, 2 tsp sea salt, 1 tsp ground black pepper and the paprika, and sprinkle over the parsnips. Toss well, then lay the parsnips out on one large baking tray (or two small ones), with lots of space between them. Roast for 15 mins, turn them over, then roast for another 20-25 mins until golden and crunchy.

Spicy cauliflower pilau

Ingredients

- 225g cauliflower florets (not the stalk)

- 3 cloves

- ½ cinnamon stick

- ½ tsp turmeric

- 6 curry leaves

Directions

- STEP 1

Put the cauliflower florets in a food processor and pulse to make grains the size of rice. Tip into a microwaveable bowl and stir in the cloves, cinnamon stick, turmeric and curry leaves.

• STEP 2

Mix well, cover with cling film, pierce and microwave on High for 3 mins. Fluff up with a fork and serve.

Wilted spinach with nutmeg & garlic

Ingredients

• 1-2 tbsp olive oil

• 4 garlic cloves, chopped

• 500g bag baby spinach leaves

* 1 nutmeg

Directions

* STEP 1

Heat the oil in a large wok, add the garlic and stir-fry until it starts to soften. Add the spinach in big handfuls, putting more in the pan as it wilts.

* STEP 2

Grate in about an eighth of a nutmeg and mix well. Serve straight away.

Clementine & Port spiced cranberry sauce

Ingredients

* 450g cranberries, thawed if frozen

* grated zest and juice 2 clementines

* 2 tbsp port

* 1 cinnamon stick

* 3 cardamom pods, bruised

* 75g sugar

Directions

* STEP 1

Put all the Ingredients in a saucepan and stir over a gentle heat until the sugar has dissolved. Increase the heat, cover and simmer for 5 mins until the cranberries have burst and the sauce has thickened. Transfer to a bowl and leave to cool, then remove the cinnamon and cardamom.

Salted caramel parsnips

Ingredients

- 1kg parsnip, peeled

- 3 tbsp rapeseed oil

- 50g golden caster sugar

- large knob of butter

- 1 tsp sea salt

Directions

- STEP 1

Heat oven to 220C/200C fan/gas 7. Halve the parsnips, then cut the thicker end in two lengthways. Boil for 5 mins, then drain well and leave to steam-dry for a few mins. Meanwhile, pour the oil into a shallow roasting tin or a lipped baking tray and heat in the oven for 3 mins.

• STEP 2

Remove the tin from the oven and carefully add the parsnips to the hot oil. Turn them to coat, and make sure they aren't overcrowded (otherwise they won't crisp up). Roast for 30-35 mins or until golden and crisp, turning them halfway through the cooking time.

• STEP 3

About 10 mins before the parsnips are ready, tip the sugar and 2 tbsp water into a small frying pan. Heat very gently until the sugar has dissolved. Turn up the heat and bring the liquid to the boil.

Measure 3½ tbsp cold water into a jug. Keep swirling the pan around until the sugar reaches a rich, dark-reddish caramel colour, then remove from the heat. Stand well back and add the water (it will splutter!). Return to the heat, add the butter and the salt, and stir to remove any lumps. The caramel should be runny, so add a splash more water if needed. Pile the parsnips into a serving dish, then drizzle over the salted caramel.

Tomato, watermelon & feta salad with mint dressing

Ingredients

• 2 tbsp olive oil

• 1 tbsp red wine vinegar

- ¼ tsp chilli flakes

- 2 tbsp chopped mint

- 4 tomatoes, chopped

- 500g/1lb 2oz watermelon, cut into chunks

- 200g pack feta cheese, crumbled

Directions

- STEP 1

Make the dressing by mixing the oil, vinegar, chilli flakes and mint with some seasoning.

- STEP 2

Put the tomatoes and watermelon in a bowl. Pour over the dressing and leave to stand for 10 mins to allow the fruit to get really juicy. Gently stir through the feta, then serve.

Pickled carrot & mooli

Ingredients

* ½ mooli (about 225g), peeled and cut into matchsticks

* 1 carrot, cut into matchsticks

* 3 tbsp rice vinegar

* 3 tbsp caster sugar

Directions

• STEP 1

Pack the mooli and carrot into a jar or small bowl. Mix together 250ml warm water and the vinegar, sugar and 2 tbsp sea salt until the sugar and salt have dissolved.

• STEP 2

Pour the mixture over the mooli and carrot. Pop on the jar lid or cover the bowl with cling film and leave for at least 1 hr or up to 3 days. Will keep for 1 week in the fridge.

Spiced braised red cabbage

Ingredients

• 1 star anise

- 1 cinnamon stick

- 5 cardamom pods

- 1 small red cabbage (about 900g)

- 1 garlic clove

- 2 large onions, chopped

- 1 Bramley apple, peeled, cored and finely chopped

- 3 tbsp brown sugar

- 3 tbsp red wine vinegar

- 25g butter

Directions

- STEP 1

Heat oven to 150C/130C fan/gas 2. Put the star anise, cinnamon stick and cardamom pods in the centre of a small square of muslin, and tie the ends together to make a bag. Put the spice bag in a medium flameproof casserole dish.

- STEP 2

Remove any wilted or tough outer leaves from the cabbage. Cut it into quarters, then remove and discard the core. Shred the cabbage finely and layer up in the dish with the garlic, onions, apple and brown sugar.

- STEP 3

Spoon over the vinegar and dot the top with the butter. Cover with a lid and cook for 21/2-3 hrs, stirring twice during cooking – the cabbage should be tender but not mushy. Remove the spice bag and serve.

Monitoring symptoms and making adjustments to your diet

Diarrhea and bloating are perhaps the most common side effects individuals experience when eliminating gluten from their diets. There are several different ways you can stop or reduce these symptoms.

1. Eliminate Alcohol, Caffeine, and Sugar from Your Diet

Consuming these requires your digestive system to work hard. Temporarily removing these consumables from your diet (including carbs that turn into sugar) will give your digestive system a much-needed break while it's trying to adjust to the removal of gluten from your diet.

2. Consume More Wholefoods

Processed foods are likely to have hidden sources of gluten in them and tend to be hard for your digestive system to process. Fresh fruits and vegetables, lean proteins, nuts, and grains are more easily digestible, which will put less pressure on your already vulnerable digestive system.

3. Temporarily Eliminate Dairy from Your Diet

Dairy is another food product that is hard for your digestive system to process. You may want to reintroduce dairy into your diet, provided you don't also discover that you're lactose intolerant now that you've removed gluten from your diet.

4. Take the Proper Supplements

Probiotics help grow the good bacteria in your gut. You can ingest these by consuming food high in probiotics like kimchi or kombucha. Buying these in supplements format is also a great option. Enzyme-rich supplements or vitamins should also be added to your list as they help your body break down the food you consume making it easier for absorption.

Both can create more stability in your gastrointestinal tract. Adults don't generally get enough magnesium in their diets. This deficiency can result in muscle cramps when you're withdrawing from gluten-rich grains.

5. Increase Your Water Intake

Removing gluten products from your diet can cause a drop in insulin levels, resulting in muscle cramps, nausea, and dizziness. Increasing your hydration levels during the earliest days after removing gluten from your diet will help you minimize these side effects.

6. Increase Your Consumption of Sodium and Iodine

As processed food are high in sodium, eliminating these from your diet will result in a drop in your salt intake. Sodium is critical to reducing cramping and cloudy thoughts that come with a drop in insulin level and dehydration.

Intentionally supplementing your diet with sodium and iodine should alleviate some of your gluten withdrawal symptoms.

If your withdrawal symptoms don't subside within a week or two, then you might not have entirely eliminated all gluten-containing foods from your diet. You may also find that cross-contamination has occurred.

Long-term benefits of a low FODMAP, high fiber, and gluten-free lifestyle

Switching to a low FODMAP, high fiber, and gluten-free lifestyle can bring about a lot of long-term benefits for your overall health. When you cut down on fermentable carbs like FODMAPs, it often eases symptoms linked to irritable bowel syndrome (IBS), such as bloating and stomach discomfort. This kind of diet helps your digestion work better and lets your body absorb nutrients more efficiently.

Plus, a fiber-rich diet keeps your bowel movements regular, lowers cholesterol levels, and supports maintaining a healthy weight. It also lowers the risk of chronic diseases like heart disease, diabetes, and certain cancers. Going gluten-free can be especially helpful for people with gluten sensitivity or celiac disease, reducing inflammation and promoting better gut health.

In the long run, sticking to these healthy eating habits doesn't just benefit your physical health — it can also boost your mental well-being by reducing discomfort and improving your overall quality of life. Making these changes to your diet can lead to lasting improvements in your health, making it a worthwhile choice for your future well-being.